OKLAHOMA PRIDE

Working Together for the Well-being of all Oklahomans

Edited by

DR. GARY E RASKOB

With a foreword by

GENE RAINBOLT

And contributions by

SHARON NEUWALD

SHAUNA LAWYER STRUBY

MARVIN SMITH

© 2021 Full Circle Press
All rights reserved. Reprint with permission

Published by Full Circle Press
a division of Full Circle Bookstore LLC
1900 North West Expressway,
Oklahoma City, Oklahoma 73118

Dr. Gary Raskob, editor

Dr. Sharon Neuwald, lead writer,
with contributions by Shauna Lawyer Struby
and Marvin Smith

Illustrations provided by the School of Visual Art,
Weitzenhoffer Family College of Fine Arts,
University of Oklahoma

The Seed Sower © 2000 Paul Moore

Cover: *Oklahoma Pride* © 2021 Greg Burns

Book, text, and jacket design by
Carl Brune

Printed in Canada

First edition. First printing

ISBN 978-0-9858651-7-7

CONTENTS

Foreword

I treasure my Oklahoma heritage and speak with gratitude about my Oklahoma roots. I care about the people of Oklahoma.

I have lived long enough to witness their struggles. Living through the Great Depression impacted me deeply. Many farmers lost their livelihoods. I saw the effects of the "Dust Bowl" landscape so powerfully described in the *Grapes of Wrath*. I understand the lyric written by Woody Guthrie in his song *Tom Joad*. "Wherever little children are hungry and cry, wherever people ain't free. Wherever men are fightin' for their rights, that's where I'm a-gonna be." I identify myself as the mythical cousin of Tom Joad.

Out of the despair of the 1930s came strong leadership. In 1932, it took the form of new institutions and programs such as Social Security, the Civilian Conservation Corps and the formation of the Federal Deposit Insurance Corporation (FDIC). Today these very same entities stand as the foundations of our nation's courageous act.

I believe Oklahoma is at a similar crossroads. We lag behind the rest of the nation in the educational progress of our children, the financial security of our families, the very health of our children and adults, and equal opportunities for each and every citizen regardless of their gender identity, cultural identity, perceived skin color, religion, education, choice of partner, or economic status.

We have higher rates of people uninsured, infant mortality, and death from heart disease than anywhere else in the country. We have families living in poverty. Oklahoma has the highest rate of incarceration in the United States and the world. This comes at the same time that Oklahoma students are at the bottom in completing high school and college degrees.

Throughout my life, I have seen the vacuum created by the absence of emboldened leadership and public support. For me it is simple: "If you can get people to work together you can get more done." It is about mobilizing actions at the community and state levels to nurture those who call Oklahoma home.

Oklahoma Pride: Working Together for the Well-being of All Oklahomans is my love letter to the state imploring us to take the needed actions to improve the lives of our residents.

I ask you to join me in this call to action.

GENE RAINBOLT

Introduction

We are pleased to present *Oklahoma Pride: Working Together for the Well-being of All Oklahomans*. Oklahoma Pride speaks to the joy we have in the way our communities respond to critical situations with an outpouring of strength, support and kindness. This book calls on us to apply these same values to improve the well-being of Oklahomans for years to come. This book was written in the middle of the COVID-19 pandemic, which forced profound changes in all of our lives. The challenges facing champions of this book were the need to redirect efforts towards a host of issues involved in tackling this virus. These efforts caused a delay in the final publication of this book which we are proud to finally present to you.

The concerns magnified during the pandemic mirror conditions described in this book. The artists' illustrations point to poor outcomes along many dimensions for low-income individuals and those in minority groups. These conditions speak to the need for individuals to not only have better health care, but also adequate income, housing and additional work and educational opportunities. In this way all individuals may realize their best possible health.

In so many areas, we see situations that threaten the health, education and financial strength of our residents. Despite many past initiatives, Oklahoma still ranks near the bottom of the nation on key health and social measures. Here are but a few examples illustrating the size of the state's problems. Oklahoma ranks as one of the bottom five states in the nation on infant and cancer deaths. Oklahoma also scores a D or F on infant mortality and teen birth rates, as well as the percent of the population who are uninsured or living in poverty.[1][2][3]

Yet these low marks did not always represent where Oklahoma stood. In 1990, Oklahoma ranked 32nd in overall health. By 2009, Oklahoma had bottomed out, declining to 49th in the nation. Yet the state through determination and strategic action improved over several years from this second worst national ranking to being 43rd in 2017 but then declining to 46th in 2019.[4] Yet are we okay with settling for 46th in the nation? Why has Oklahoma lost ground on critical measures affecting the health of our residents? We know we can do better and must. With that in mind, we asked community

In 1990, Oklahoma ranked 32nd in overall health; by 2019, the state had declined to 46th in the country, dropping 14 points over the past 30 years.

leaders to come together to better understand factors affecting Oklahomans' health and offer a way to communicate both concerns and recommended solutions to the public.

We wanted to take a fresh look at these health issues. What distinguishes this work from others is the partnership forged with the University of Oklahoma School of Visual Arts within the Weitzenhoffer Family College of Fine Arts. Students in that program demonstrated their creativity and talent to illustrate where Oklahoma stands now and what it will need to do to create a healthier future. Hearing from new younger voices is critical, since it will ultimately be their generation's responsibility to convert this vision into reality for our state. For us, Oklahoma Pride is the culmination of these students' research and imagination.

Oklahoma Pride is organized into three sections. The indicators under *The State of our Health* measure conditions that affect the length and quality of Oklahoma residents' lives. The second section, *The Risks We Take*, include measures that describe behaviors that affect these results. The third section, *Conditions Affecting Our Health,* looks at poverty, education and health insurance status to predict how well and how long people live.[5][6] This book is extensively referenced to original sources of data and research. While current at the time of writing, some of these sources may have been updated during the production of the book. We encourage the reader to explore the sources listed and continue to learn about the state of Oklahoma's health and well being. We believe the solutions to the challenges facing Oklahoma will be most effective if they are grounded in the evidence from sound public health and social science research.

The history of Oklahoma throughout its 114 years of statehood is marked not only by hard times, but by determination and a spirit of self-reliance. While necessary for survival, this legacy of independence sometimes holds us back. We wonder how Oklahoma's history would have unfolded if there had been greater cooperative efforts around reaching the lofty goals described in this book.[7]

It is with this understanding that we present *Oklahoma Pride,* identifying actions necessary for Oklahomans to prosper in the 21st century. It is essential for us to work together with many partners inside and outside of health care to improve on the conditions described in this book. Our two-year engagement involved experts in the areas of public health, journalism, business and the arts. We drew upon the talent and creativity of college students, our next generation of leaders. Through their eyes, we see portraits of despair if we continue on the same path and illustrations of joy if we act on behalf of a vision of what this state can be—a place which emphasizes the health of all Oklahomans.

We hope as you take in these recommendations, that you demand action from our state and community leaders. By working together, we can carry out the students' dreams to dramatically improve the long-term health and well-being of our residents. We can think of no greater endeavor.

THE STATE
OF OUR HEALTH

I never got to hold you, or bounce you on my lap. I never got to read to you, or watch you as you nap. You slipped away so quickly before I said your name. And I want the world to know, I loved you just the same.[1]

~ A PETERSON

INFANT MORTALITY

This is the expression of anguish by parents who lose their infants, a sorrow where words seem inadequate to describe their pain. The infant mortality rate (IMR) is the number of infants who die before one year of age for every 1,000 live births, an important measure since it is considered a marker for the overall health in our society.[2][3]

While Oklahoma's IMR rate has decreased by 17 percent since 2007, the state still ranks as the 3rd worst state in the nation with an IMR of 7.6 per 1,000 live births, higher than the overall country's rate of 5.8.[4][5][6]

Two babies die every hour in the USA. Every 12 hours a woman dies as a result of complications from pregnancy. Oklahoma is the 3rd worst state in the nation for its infant mortality rate. For 2017 Oklahoma received an F in the "State of the State's Health" report card.

Here we see the impact of so many infants dying in our state. It is row after row of high chairs hovering around small burial places. The collection of infant graves is heartbreaking. The artists mirror the pain that parents must feel at the loss of someone so beloved whom they will never get to know.

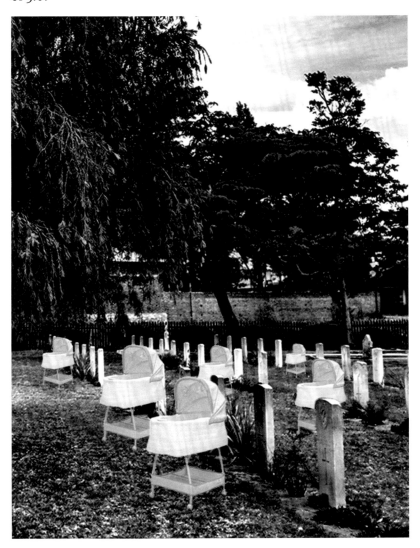

On this measure, for 2017, Oklahoma received an F grade in the "State of the State's Health" report card.[7]

Its frequency is disturbing. Two babies die every hour in the U.S.A. Every 12 hours a woman dies as a result of complications from pregnancy. For affected families, it is difficult to forget and move on.[8]

* * * * * * * * *

Our artists clearly show us the importance of good prenatal and post-partum care. The state through its "Preparing for a Lifetime, Its Everyone's Responsibility" campaign identifies how mothers can keep themselves and their babies healthy. Personal actions are important and include mothers remaining healthy between pregnancies, eliminating smoking and alcohol use, taking prenatal vitamins, including folic acid, and establishing a safe sleep environment for the baby. These behaviors are key, having been shown to improve birth outcomes and minimize infant deaths or disabilities.[9][10][11][12][13]

There are also policies and programs that can improve pregnancy outcomes in the long term. The state should adopt policies that increase access to care, before, during and after pregnancies, expand health insurance coverage, fund training to increase the number of health care providers and locate medical practices in maternity care deserts.[14][15][16][17] Actions that address racial/ethnic differences in infant mortality need to consider conditions in poor communities: education gaps, poverty, transportation limits, poor nutrition, unsafe and unaffordable housing and few safe play areas.[18][19][20] Specific programs can make a difference like parenting/healthy relationship services, home visitation and quality child care.[21][22][23][24][25] Community models tailored to racial and ethnic traditions have been shown to improve birth outcomes for minority populations.[26][27]

Acting on these recommendations will ensure infant mortality continues to decline in Oklahoma. Let's support these changes to sustain the progress we have made so far.

Parents who have lost a child have increased risk of guilt, depression, heart attacks, post-traumatic stress disorder and psychiatric hospitalizations.[28] The leading causes of infant deaths are birth defects, preterm births, pregnancy complications, sudden infant death syndrome and injuries like suffocation.[29] [30] [31] [32] [33] A higher risk of infant mortality is associated with single parents and those under the age of 20 or over 40.[34] [35] [36] [37]

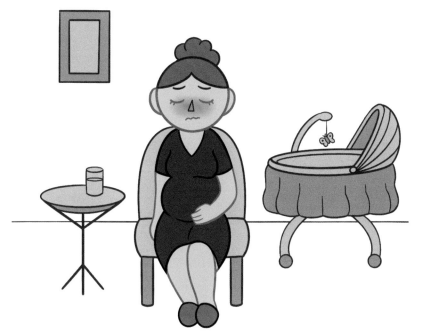

Here is a woman who does not feel well. Does she fear the consequences of being poor and uninsured? How will she get good prenatal care? Will her care come too late, putting herself and her baby at risk? Could it lead to another infant death in the state?

Of great importance are the racial differences: infant mortality rates for Black or African Americans are more than twice as high and 1.9 times as high for American Indians as they are for white infants.[38] While medical factors play a role, racial and ethnic differences can also be attributed to growing up in communities with high levels of poverty and inadequate health care. These negative environmental conditions can affect not only the mother but also the baby during pregnancy.[39] [40] [41] [42]

Here is a future where regular doctor visits help the mother get the care she needs. Instead of a field of dead babies, we see what it takes to get good care. Prenatal vitamins and needed tests, like sonograms, are in full display as part of a comprehensive package of early ongoing prenatal services.

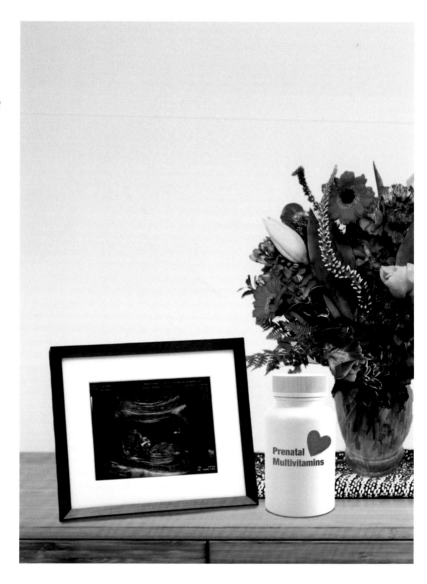

The artists' vision is to see that all women in Oklahoma get early, adequate prenatal care to maximize the likelihood of healthy births. Prenatal care is more likely to be effective if women begin care during the first three months of pregnancy with continued visits until delivery. Yet, in 2018, only 70 percent of Oklahoman women began prenatal care in the first 3 months.[43]

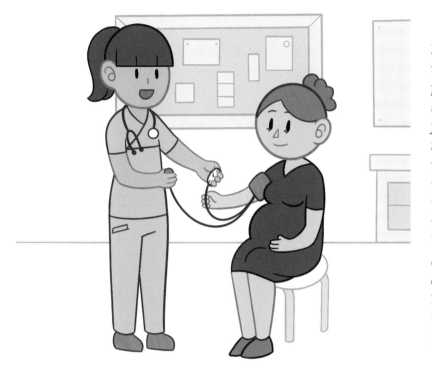

Now this woman is getting needed prenatal care, setting the stage for a healthy birth. Students imagine what a comfort it is for this woman to now have health insurance, allowing her to find a good doctor to manage her care. The stress has left her face since she knows she is in good hands.

Infant mortality and life expectancy are reasonable indicators of general well-being in a society.[44]

~ P.J. O'ROURKE
JOURNALIST AND
POLITICAL SATIRIST

When someone has cancer the whole family and everyone who loves them does too.[1]

CANCER DEATHS

The quote on the preceding page expresses the widespread repercussions cancer has on both patients and their families. Oklahomans have a right to worry since Oklahoma ranks as the 4th worst state in the nation for cancer deaths with 178.1 overall deaths per 100,000 residents compared to a national rate of 149.1 per 100,000 individuals.[2] [3] This concern is in the context of cancer being the second leading cause of death in the United States, exceeded only by heart disease. One of every 4 deaths in the United States is due to cancer. [4]

The artists represent the anguish involved in being faced with cancer and reflects a surreal experience during a cancer diagnosis.

Oklahoma ranks as the 4th worst state in the nation for cancer deaths.

An expressionless woman, her body ravaged by cancer, symbolizes the mind-numbing moment when the reality of her situation becomes clear. Cancer can be silent and invisible until it breaks through as a debilitating force on the body, negatively affecting a person's health. This image also suggests a dire prognosis of an advanced stage of cancer, and perhaps reflects the bleak outcome for the over 8,400 Oklahomans that died of cancer in 2020.[5]

9

The artists offer an optimistic vision where there is widespread utilization of screenings and early detection to significantly lower cancer rates in Oklahoma.

Age, weight, exposure to carcinogens, and genetics can increase the risk of developing cancer.[6] Across all types of cancer, smoking causes 19 percent, and a combination of being overweight, physical inactivity, excess alcohol consumption, and poor nutrition cause 18 percent.[7] While there is no universal cure, lifestyle changes can lower cancer death rates. Quitting smoking at any age lowers the risk of developing cancer. Physical activity, maintaining a healthy weight, limiting alcohol use, and avoiding excessive sun exposure are linked to lower risks of certain cancers. Following recommended schedules for screenings—especially for breast, colon, cervical, and prostate cancers—can improve outcomes by detecting the disease at earlier stages. Regular screenings and the human papillomavirus (HPV) vaccine can prevent more than 90% of cervical cancer while the hepatitis B vaccine can help reduce the risk of liver cancer.[8][9]

Addressing the widening gap between those with higher standards of living and those in poverty can improve cancer death rates. Racial and ethnic differences in cancer rates reflect the excessive numbers in poverty as well as disparities in the quality of health care received.[10] Lack of health insurance prevents many individuals from receiving the best cancer prevention, early detection and care resulting in a greater chance of an advanced-stage cancer diagnosis. Expanding the number of insured individuals in Oklahoma as well as increasing access for low-income individuals and minorities to all levels of services can help reduce disparities in cancer for these groups.[11][12][13]

Individual and community actions, coupled with policy changes, will continue Oklahoma's progress toward reducing cancer death rates.[14] These recommended strategies, by preventing and improving cancer outcomes, will not only impact the lives of affected Oklahomans but will contribute to the overall long-term well-being of its residents, hopefully resulting in less fear associated with this disease.

By following the recommendations of medical experts for regular screenings, any cancer that may develop is more likely to be diagnosed early, with treatment having a better chance of success, and the woman much more likely to live a longer and healthier life. By showing the positive side of early screening, detection and treatment, the artists connect us to the declining cancer death rate in the U.S. that's occurred over the past 25 years.[15][16]

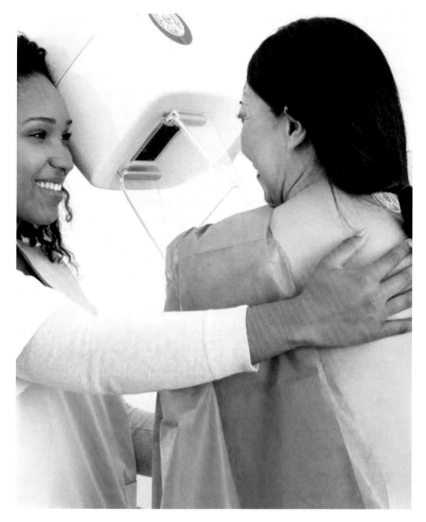

Here is a visualization of what occurs when a patient is aware and acts based on knowledge about the best ways to prevent and treat cancer. The artists portray a woman, taking charge of her care, at a mammography appointment, suggesting the screening is part of a regular preventive healthcare regimen.

Many cancer deaths could be prevented by following a balanced diet, staying physically active, eliminating tobacco use, following routine cancer screening recommendations, obtaining preventative vaccinations, and avoiding exposure to the sun or indoor tanning devices.[17]

~ DAVID DUDE
AMERICAN CANCER SOCIETY IN OKLAHOMA

CANCER DEATHS

I remember thinking that my kids would be better off if I wasn't here. I was homeless, jobless! I felt like someone else would be better able to take care of them.[1]

~ NANCY, SUICIDE SURVIVOR

SUICIDE DEATH RATE

Oklahoma is the 9th highest state in the nation for suicide; At 20.5 per 100,000 individuals, the State's rate is 38.5 percent higher than the national rate at 14.5 per 100,000.[2] In addition to the devastating human toll, the financial consequences are huge. For 2010, it cost Oklahoma more than $778 million in combined lifetime medical expenses and work loss. This averaged more than $1.2 million per suicide death.[3]

The students present poignant images of the struggles individuals face as well as the disturbing and destructive consequences of suicide.

Oklahoma is the 9th worst state in the nation for suicide.

Nooses hang silently from playground equipment, serving as powerful symbols of the loneliness faced by those committing suicide and the magnitude of this problem. We carry the loss of our children and adults with a heavy heart. We berate ourselves for looking away from their struggles. This equipment could be in a park, suggesting suicide is something we cannot ignore. We have to admit suicide is society's dilemma— not an "over there"— or "someone else's" problem.

The students show us suicide is not the inevitable outcome for someone feeling despondent. It will take a variety of approaches to lower Oklahoma's suicide rate.

We need to support screening and suicide awareness training to ensure frontline workers learn how to effectively respond to potential suicide situations.[4] [5] We must strengthen insurance coverage for treatment of mental health conditions. There needs to be much more clinical care in our state using proven effective forms of therapy for the treatment of mental and substance abuse disorders. It is important to have services that work with families to develop effective coping, parenting and problem solving skills as well as youth development and community engagement programs.[6] Firearm and drug safety programs as well as policies that lower excess alcohol use are important strategies for reducing access to the means of suicide and its contributing factors. The impact of poverty cannot be ignored. We must strengthen economic supports for families by looking at ways to increase their financial security as well as opportunities for more stable housing arrangements.[7] Higher educational attainment and better job opportunities need to be part of this multi-pronged approach in communities with concentrated poverty.[8] [9]

These actions hold the best promise for reversing the rising tide of suicide in Oklahoma. Early identification and treatment, connections to needed resources, local engagement and improvement in the social and economic conditions of low-income communities are the actions needed to achieve a long lasting impact.

There are groups that are at high risk of suicide. Men in Oklahoma commit suicide at more than 3 times the rate as women. Whites and Native Americans have the highest rates of suicide in the nation and the state.[10] [11] In Oklahoma, suicides by Oklahoman youth have increased 103 percent since 2007 compared to a 42 percent increase nationally.[12] LGBTQ youth and adults often face isolation and victimization, making them a high risk for suicidal behaviors.[13]

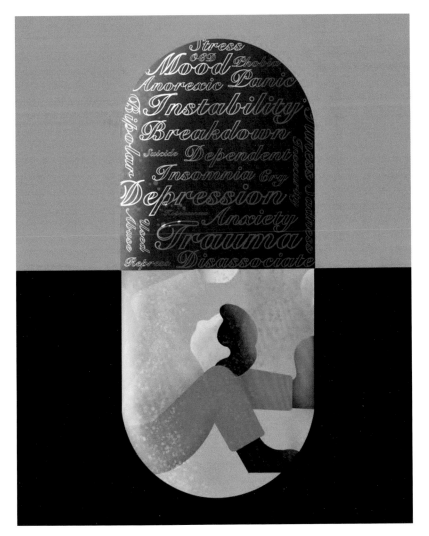

Look how this boy is crushed by the weight of his situation. The artists show him trying to free himself, yet trapped in addiction and mental illness. Facing this struggle, the students, portray this boy as a fighter, yet stuck in what we can only imagine is his own despair.

There is no single cause for suicides. Physical and psychological difficulties, a history of depression, trauma and violence, access to lethal methods and lack of supports are all contributing factors.[14] [15] Warning signs that someone is contemplating suicide include mood changes, discussions about killing oneself, increased use of alcohol and drugs as well as withdrawal and isolation.[16]

SUICIDE DEATH RATE

The students understand the importance of connections and receiving needed treatment to overcome the sense of hopelessness and despair that can lead to suicide. Their solutions call out to let these troubled individuals know they are not alone; we hear their pleas and are there to help.

To prevent suicides, the artists urge us to begin by having a conversation. It takes courage to reach out to others. How comforting that this man has found someone who cares for him. Will he now be able to share his deepest feelings since there is no shame, no judgment about his mental illness? Connections are the solution offering support and treatment for this young man.

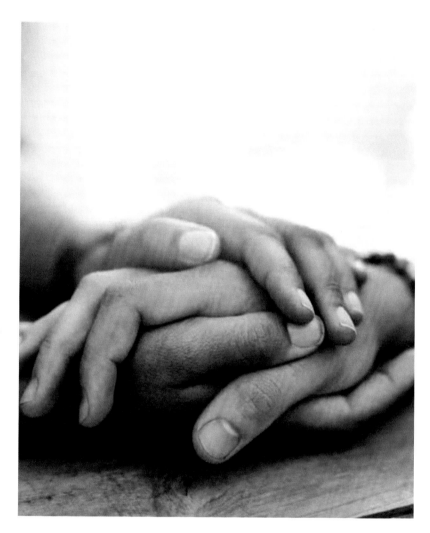

SUICIDE DEATH RATE

16

Mental health or substance abuse disorders are the most significant risk factors for suicidal behavior.[17] [18] Barriers to health care, especially treatment services, are a problem, and many individuals feel a stigma to getting help.[19] Suicide has increased most rapidly in areas with less resources: rural settings and counties with high poverty levels, lower educational achievement and higher unemployment rates.[20] [21] [22] [23] [24]

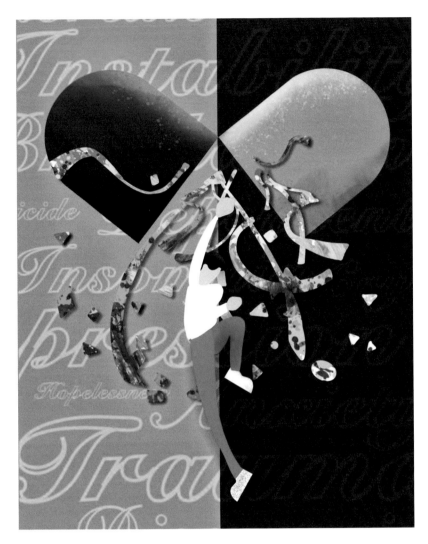

The artists express the joy and gratitude this boy experiences now that he is free from the bondage and pain of mental illness. He is feeling alive again since he has found the help he needs. Now, resources are readily available for his mental health care. The artists imagine him hitting his stride and moving forward with anticipation and optimism.

Suicide is not inevitable for anyone. By starting the conversation, providing support, and directing help to those who need it, we can prevent suicides and save lives.[25]

SUICIDE PREVENTION LIFELINE

I felt hopeless. There was no way out. At the age of 18, I was arrested around 14 times, and I overdosed, which almost cost my life.[1]

~ CHRISTOPHER DICKIE

ADDICTION AND DRUG DEATHS

Christopher's life spiraled out of control when, at age 15, he started using drugs. Over the next five years he failed to graduate from high school, lost job after job, had multiple arrests, and in one year, overdosed before finally recovering with treatment for his addiction.

Nearly 700 Oklahomans die each year from an overdose.[2] In 2020, Oklahoma ranked 23rd in the nation for drug deaths, with 18.8 deaths per 100,000 residents.[3][4][5] The costs of substance abuse disorders to Oklahoma are estimated at nearly $7.2 billion annually, an amount equal to about $1,900 a year for every Oklahoma resident.[6]

Nearly 700 Oklahomans die each year from an overdose. The costs of substance abuse disorders to Oklahoma are estimated at nearly $7.2 billion annually, an amount equal to about $1,900 a year for every Oklahoma resident.

Set against the backdrop of a stark black background, the artists show candles with prescription labels, syringes, and spoons used for reducing drugs to an injectable form. What starts with a doctor's prescription for drugs like opioids, quickly progresses to nonmedical use, spiraling out of control with drug dependence and abuse the result.

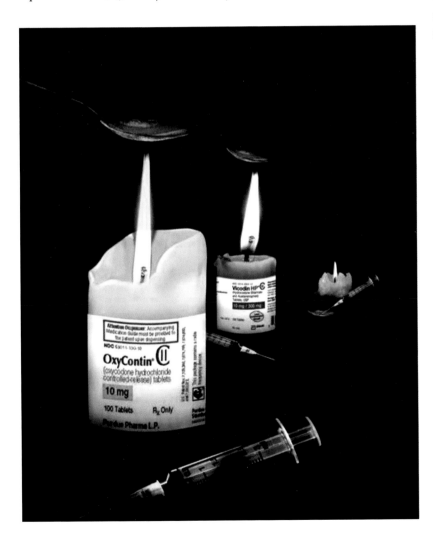

The artists' plea to reduce nonmedical use of prescription drugs is on the right path. Thankfully, the state of Oklahoma recognized the need to reduce addiction and drug overdose deaths, and in 2017 created the Oklahoma Commission on Opioid Abuse (OCOA). While their efforts have resulted in declining fatal prescription drug overdoses, much still needs to be done. Additionally, the switch to illegal drugs is a persistent problem that emphasizes an ongoing need for addiction treatment, resources, and research.[7][8]

OCOA's 2019 report includes a range of recommendations such as amending Oklahoma's parity law to ensure health insurance companies cover addiction treatment on par with other chronic medical conditions such as heart disease and diabetes. Given the fact that Oklahoma has the second highest number of uninsured people in the nation, it is also critical that expanded Medicaid coverage increase access to addiction treatment.[9]

Additional recommendations from OCOA and others focus on expanding effective addiction treatment options that include a multi-disciplinary approach utilizing individual treatment plans, therapy, use of medication assisted treatment (MAT) if needed, crisis intervention, outpatient services and more.[10][11][12] In addition, substance abuse screening and early intervention protocols should be part of primary care physician visits as is done for chronic conditions like diabetes. Early responders, middle and high school students, coaches and athletes need to learn about the dangers of addiction and how to intervene early. Given the strong links between adverse childhood experiences (ACEs) and illegal drug use in adulthood, the state should support programs that prevent ACEs such as parent engagement services, teen pregnancy prevention, violence prevention, home visitation programs for pregnant women, and income supports for at-risk low-income residents. We need to encourage legislators to adequately fund and reform eligibility for drug courts which help participants receive treatment as an alternative to incarceration. [13] [14] We need to encourage legislators to adequately fund drug courts which helps participants receive treatment as an alternative to incarceration.[15]

These recommendations will produce a significant and long-term reduction in the number of Oklahomans suffering from addiction and dying from drug overdoses. Improvements in these areas—medical, mental health and treatment communities, education, state agencies, and law enforcement, are needed to have a measurable impact on reducing substance abuse disorders and drug overdose deaths, as well as improving the overall health of Oklahomans.

Recognizing the need to rethink the way society approaches substance abuse disorders, the artists choose a preventative solution implemented by pharmacies to encourage people to clean out their medicine cabinets and safely dispose of unneeded drugs.

Understanding addiction as a chronic, relapsing brain disease rather than a choice is critical to addressing this devastating public health problem. Legal and illegal drug use involves many substances: alcohol, cocaine, hallucinogens like ecstasy, methamphetamine, heroin, and misuse of prescription drugs. Each person suffering from the disease of addiction has a different set of medical, physical, mental, and behavioral challenges.

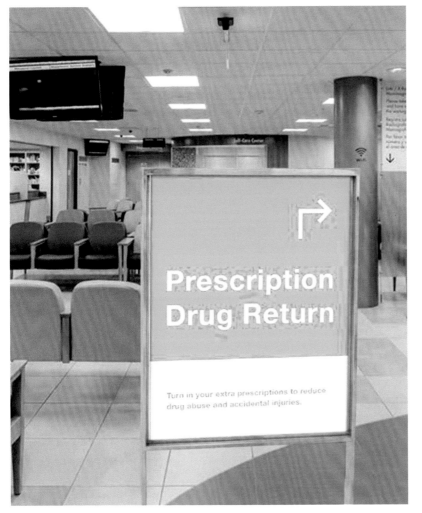

The artists select the lobby of a pharmacy to emphasize prescription drug return programs as an effective way to reduce accidental or nonmedical use of prescriptions.

ADDICTION &
DRUG DEATHS

In 2018, an estimated 43 percent of drug overdose deaths in Oklahoma involved opioids, including heroin and nonmedical use of prescription opioids such as fentanyl.[16]

Oklahoma providers wrote 79.1 opioid prescriptions for every 100 persons—compared to the average U.S. rate of 51.4 prescriptions.[17] Are these artists wondering where the pharmaceutical companies stand in acknowledging the risks of their use? The public has been exposed to advertising that minimized the addictive and dangerous nature of these drugs while doctors are inundated with marketing material. Countless individuals, families, and communities are now paying the cost in billions of dollars.

A 2017 Consumer Reports survey covering 1,006 adults found that about one-third of Americans have not cleaned out their medicine cabinets in the past year; nearly one-fifth have not done so in the past three years.[18] Pharmacies as well as hospitals, clinics, long-term-care facilities, narcotic treatment programs and city sites may accept unused medications. Disposemymeds.org is an online resource to help people find medication disposal programs at authorized facilities close to them.

Turn your wounds into wisdom.[19]

~ OPRAH WINFREY
TELEVISION PRODUCER,
ACTRESS, AUTHOR AND PHILANTHROPIST

*My recovery must come first so that
everything I love in life doesn't have
to come last.*[20]

DAILY SOBRIETY JOURNAL FOR
ADDICTION RECOVERY

THE RISKS
WE TAKE

Smoking is a habit that drains your money and kills you slowly, one puff after another. Quit smoking, start living.[1]

~ THE QUOTES MASTER

TOBACCO

Tobacco kills more Oklahomans than alcohol, auto accidents, suicides, murders and illegal drugs combined.[2] It is responsible for 7,500 deaths a year, with Oklahoma's smoking rate ranked as the 10th worst state in the nation.[3] Second-hand smoke, alone, causes 700 deaths every year.[4]

The artists illustrate a range of negative impacts tobacco use has on Oklahoma residents.

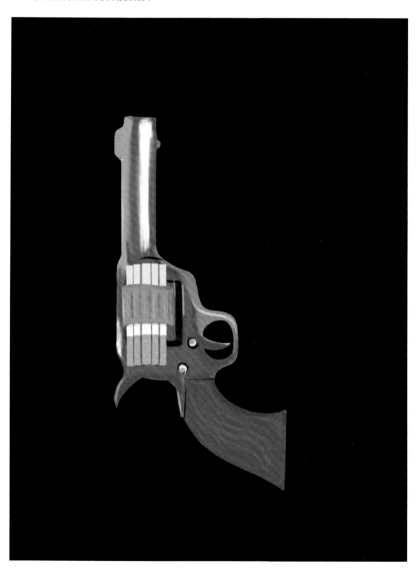

Tobacco use is responsible for 7,500 deaths a year in Oklahoma with our state's smoking rate ranked as the 10th worst state in the nation.

These artists use a gun cylinder loaded with cigarettes rather than bullets to make a poignant statement on tobacco's deadly impact. It is as if the smoker is playing cancer roulette with him or herself and those who are nearby. It is a warning to us all about the need for protections for non-smoking Oklahomans.

The artists' images depict a variety of ways to avoid the consequences of tobacco use, the leading preventable cause of death in Oklahoma. If Oklahoma reduces its smoking rate to the national rate by 2022, it is estimated there will be 150,000 fewer tobacco users in the state. [5] [6] [7]

There are proven approaches to reduce the influence of tobacco in the lives of Oklahomans. The Oklahoma Tobacco Helpline at okhelpline.org or 1-800-QUIT NOW offers a range of plans to help people quit smoking, including free patches, gums or lozenges and web-based coaching. A variety of other actions, such as those found in the Oklahoma State Plan for Tobacco Use Prevention & Cessation, approach this issue through legislation, policy changes and community action by healthcare providers, businesses, school boards, city councils, and concerned citizens. An action that has already proven successful in Oklahoma is to raise the price of tobacco products. [8] A second strategy is extending indoor smoke-free sites to include hotels and bars in Oklahoma. [9] [10] Banning menthol and flavored tobacco products would help address the increase in vaping and keep many youth from ever starting to use tobacco. [11] Cities and towns should be empowered to determine smoke-free policies by a repeal of the Oklahoma legislature's preemption law which prevents communities from taking such action. [12] A comprehensive media campaign could continue to stress the dangers of tobacco use while at the same time countering industry advertising designed to induce individuals to start. [13]

The ultimate goal should be eliminating tobacco use in Oklahoma. In this way Oklahoma would be saving both lives and dollars on the way to improving the health of all Oklahomans.

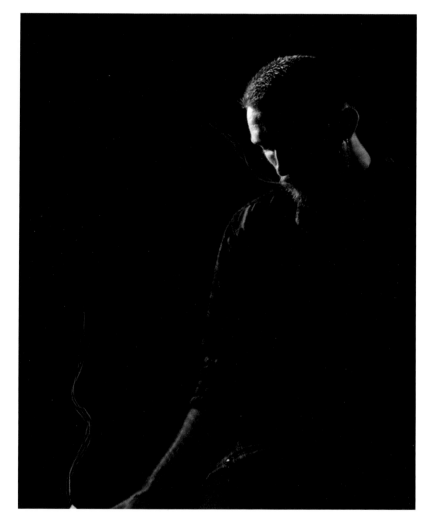

"I'm Michael. I missed my son's graduation speech because I was out smoking a cigarette."

Smoking contributes to heart disease, strokes, respiratory illnesses, and many forms of cancer.[14] Oklahoma spends more than $1.6 billion a year for medical conditions related to tobacco use.[15]

TOBACCO

29

Smoke floats across the baby in the carrier, graphically illustrating the danger of secondhand smoke to the young. For young children, secondhand smoke may consign them to asthma or frequent ear infections. [16] [17]

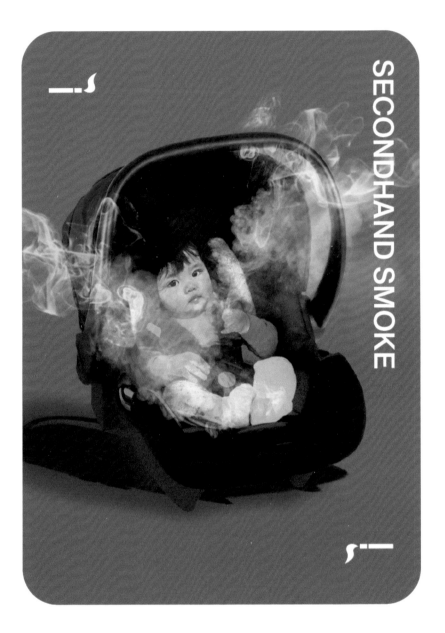

SECONDHAND SMOKE

Tobacco smoke contains more than 7,000 chemicals, including hundreds that are toxic and about 70 that can cause cancer. [18] [19]

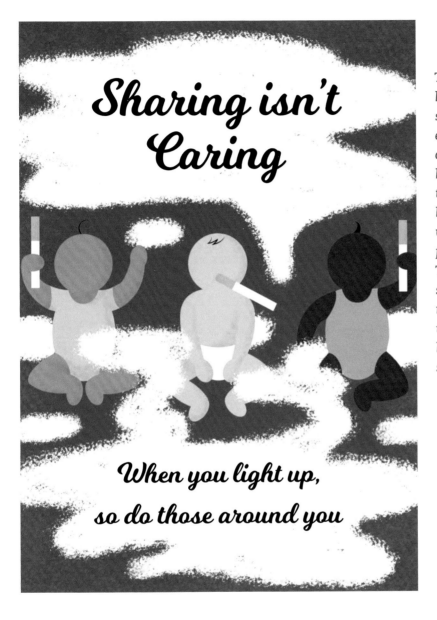

There is no risk-free level of secondhand smoke exposure; even brief encounters can be harmful to health. In this image the artists depict babies, the most vulnerable of our population, smoking. Their exposure to secondhand smoke means they will face the same dangers and harmful chemicals as smokers themselves.[20]

In this scenario, the artists choose a well-known teenage necessity—the backpack—as a symbol of the desire to fit in with friends. Combined with the vertical text, "teen smoking," the artists' message can be seen as a warning against the dangers of smoking.

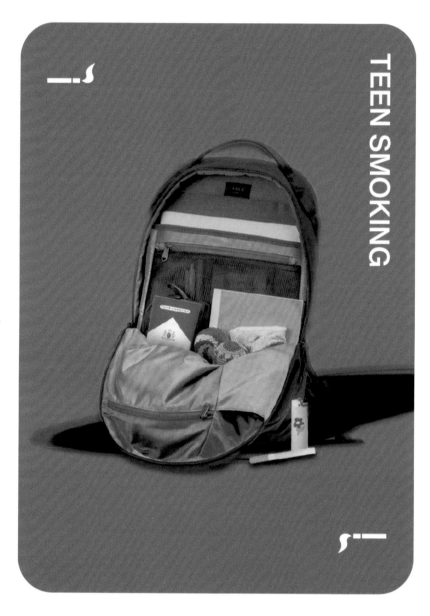

TEEN SMOKING

If cigarette smoking continues at the current rate among youth in this country, 5.6 million of today's Americans younger than 18 will die early from a smoking-related illness. [21]

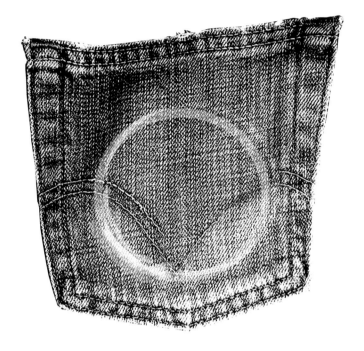

Fitting in with community traditions can be dangerous. These artists create a faded jean pocket with the imprint of a chewing tobacco tin, accompanied by a simple line of text, suggesting that we are ignoring conversations about the health risks of smokeless tobacco products.

LET'S TALK _____.

Dip, snuff and chewing tobacco are commonly used in many cities and towns in Oklahoma. Smokeless tobacco is associated with many health problems, including cancer of the mouth, esophagus, and pancreas.[22]

TOBACCO

With a nod to glamorous old movies or the teenager pulling an e-cigarette out of her purse to sneak a quick fix between classes, the artists ask a provocative question to spark much-needed conversations. All these choices in the picture contribute to the appeal of smoking.

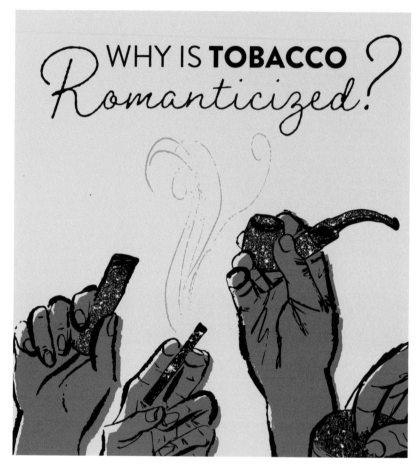

The tobacco industry is remarkably effective at marketing its products and spends billions to target specific groups of Americans, including youth and different racial and ethnic groups. The industry's latest efforts involve marketing electronic cigarettes. Oklahoma's rate of e-cigarette use is higher than the national average.[23] While e-cigarettes may be useful in helping some adult smokers cut back or quit, they are not safe for youth, young adults, pregnant women, and adults who don't use tobacco products.[24]

With an eye on a better future, the artists design imagery to inspire Oklahomans to imagine a world where tobacco is no longer a public health problem. Here is how they see it.

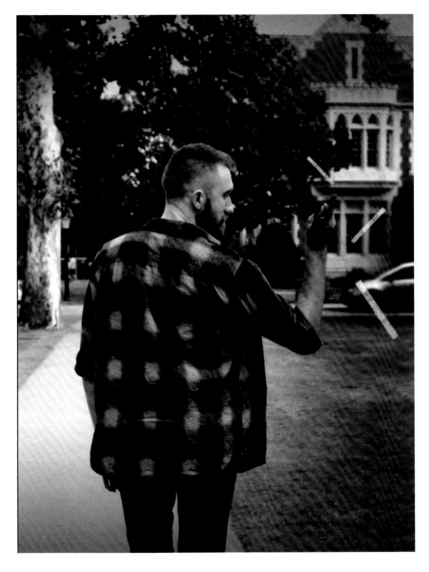

"Now, I can experience every minute of my life thanks to support that helped me quit."

TOBACCO

These artists choose a cheerful yellow backdrop and a hand clasping nicotine patches and gum—both part of nicotine replacement programs—to convey a way to quit smoking. The Oklahoma Tobacco Helpline streamlines the process with free services, easily accessible information, and non-judgmental support available online or by phone.

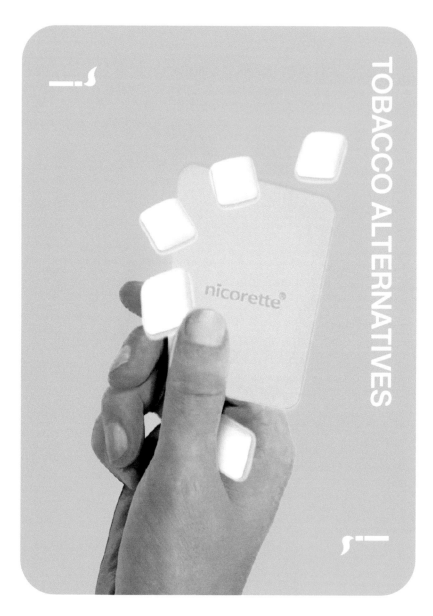

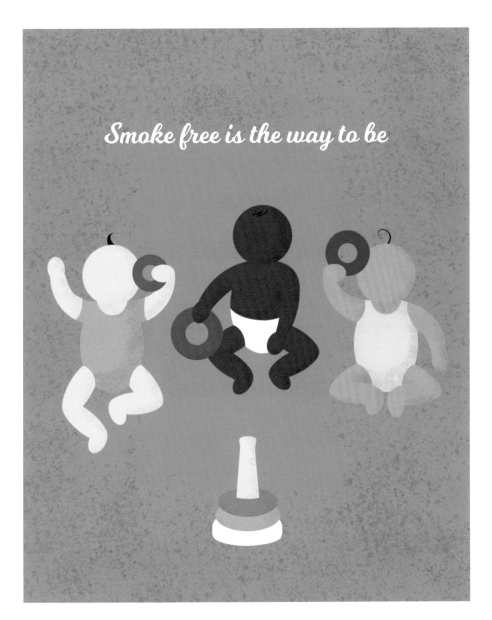

Smoke free is the way to be

Here are healthy babies sharing toys instead of cigarettes to illustrate the impact of a tobacco-free environment. Gone are the smoke-filled, smelly rooms, and nicotine-stained ceilings and walls. Now the babies can tumble around freely, breathing clean air in a healthy environment. Parents have paved a future where these babies will live healthier, longer lives.

Instead of hiding cigarettes, snuff, or e-cigarettes in a backpack the artists show a variety of tobacco products burning in an ashtray. It is a brave choice to quit, signifying a meaningful and symbolic end to an unhealthy addiction.

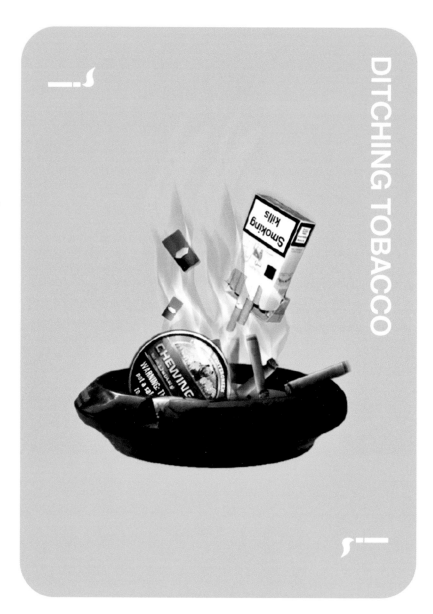

DITCHING TOBACCO

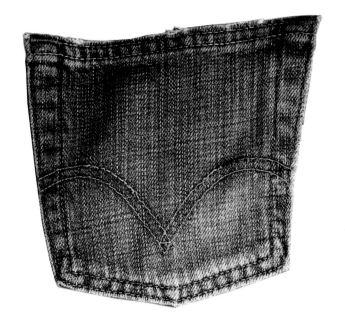

The artists depict progress in the freedom of individuals to quit dip, snuff, or other smokeless tobacco with a jean pocket absent the tin imprint. Perhaps there is a community effort to openly address and discuss the unhealthy consequences of tobacco use in all its forms as a way to help change the lives of those who are addicted.

LET'S TALK TOBACCO.

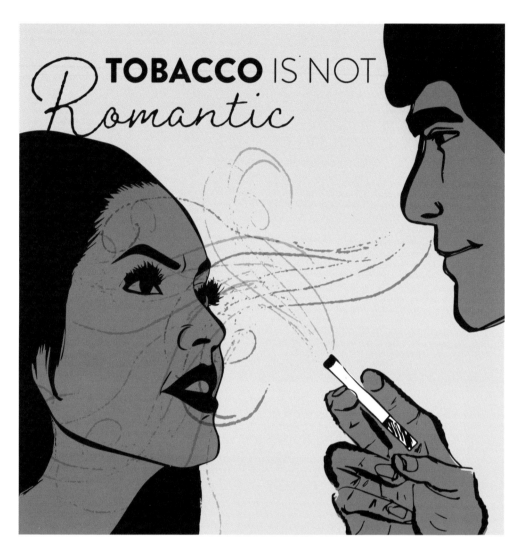

TOBACCO IS NOT *Romantic*

To represent both the unappealing nature of smoking and to counteract deceptive marketing, the artists show a woman clearly annoyed by a man smoking, who appears to be interested in her. Perhaps the artists also intend to ensure those looking for romance understand that finding the woman or man of your dreams is easier without an unhealthy habit like smoking.

You are greater than your addiction.[25]

QUOTES BY GECKO AND FLY

I quit smoking for my heart and the hearts of those I love.[26]

~ NASIA DAVOS, EX-SMOKER

The rise of childhood obesity has placed the health of an entire generation at risk.[1]

~ TOM VILSACK
GOVERNOR OF IOWA, 1999 TO 2007
SECRETARY OF AGRICULTURE, 2009–2017
CURRENT SECRETARY OF AGRICULTURE

Associated with …weight gain are increased risks in adulthood for joint problems, angina, high blood pressure, heart attacks, strokes, type 2 diabetes and, ultimately, premature death.[2]

~ JEFF SCHWEITZER
Calorie Wars: Fat, Fact and Fiction

OBESITY

As one of the nation's most pressing health problems, obesity is related to a growing number of Americans living with heart disease, high blood pressure, and diabetes. Obesity is one of the primary causes of Oklahoma's top killers—cancer and cardiovascular disease.[3] The percentage of Oklahomans who are obese—36.8 percent—has increased by more than 85 percent since 2000, making Oklahoma the 3rd worst state in the nation for adult obesity.[4] [5] [6]

The artists' illustrations in this chapter highlight the impact of obesity on individuals and call for a break in generational patterns of food preparation and consumption to create a better nutritional future. In these images, the artists present us with the two primary behaviors driving Oklahoma's obesity problem—poor eating habits and lack of exercise.

The artists picture Oklahomans rising to the challenge to improve their health and reverse course on obesity's impacts that shorten the length and quality of their lives.

The percentage of Oklahomans who are obese—36.8%—has increased by more than 85% since 2000, making Oklahoma the 3rd worst state in the nation for adult obesity.

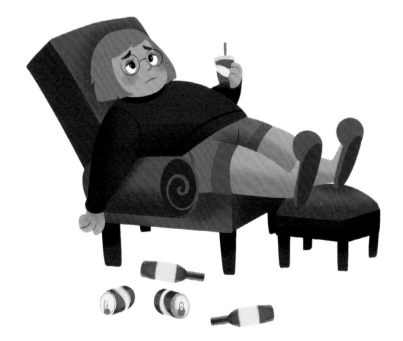

In these images, the artists imagine people who consume high-calorie beverages daily, a lifestyle that appears to bring them little joy.

The artists' hopeful vision will require targeted public health approaches for different populations in a variety of community settings such as schools, worksites and healthcare facilities. Incentives that make healthy nutritional choices and physical activity more readily available are also needed to effectively combat obesity.[7][8][9]

The workplace is an ideal setting to institute basic obesity prevention practices. Employers can do several things to help: provide in-house wellness activities, expand insurance coverage for health clubs, offer healthy snacks in vending machines and create positive incentives for breastfeeding. School-based actions can help establish healthy behaviors that children can carry with them into adulthood. They can include more physical activity during the school day, healthier food at school, hands-on teaching such as gardens at schools, and field trips to local farms or community gardens to help students establish a lifetime of healthy habits. Healthcare facilities and providers can play an important role by screening patients for physical activity during appointments and making referrals for nutrition counseling or fitness programs.[10][11]

Obesity levels tend to be higher in low-income and minority communities because their access to healthy food choices and places to be physically active are typically less available. Community strategies to promote healthy eating and encourage physical activity could include the addition of sidewalks, walking trails, and bike-share programs; more farmers markets and community gardens; as well as helping those in need apply for state and federal nutrition and other social services.[12][13]

Finally, policy changes may be needed to implement other community development strategies such as: incentivizing more physical activity in schools; price increases to discourage the consumption of unhealthy food and incentives like tax credits for private investments to maximize the development of grocery stores, better food distribution, more healthcare resources, and opportunities for physical activity in underserved communities.[14][15][16][17]

The people in our lives and the environments where we live, work, and play influence our relationship with food. Many approaches that start with individuals, family, friends and coworkers and progress to community programs are critical to the long-term reduction of Oklahoma's obesity problem, one of the leading causes of preventable death in our state.[18]

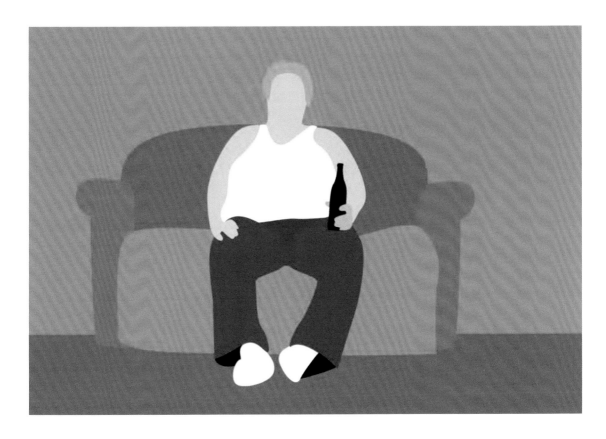

Today about 1 in 3 American adults and children are obese. If this trend continues, the rate is projected to rise to around 50 percent by 2030, magnifying the number of individuals burdened with the associated health risks.[19]

Because 34 percent of Oklahoman adults report doing no physical activity or exercise other than their jobs over a 30-day time frame, our state is ranked as the 2nd worst state in the nation for physical inactivity.[20] In 2019, less than 30 percent of Oklahoman students in 9th through 12th grade were physically active for at least 60 minutes a day; 18.1 percent of Oklahoman students in these age groups were overweight with 17.6 percent obese.[21] [22]

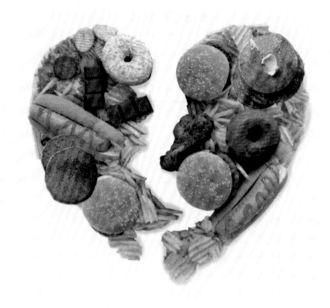

The artists portray broken hearts in two ways: A damaged heart shape comprised of fast-food meals high in saturated fats and calories, and an image of a woman, perhaps with chest pains and obviously in distress. Her face shows sadness and perhaps frustration and despair.

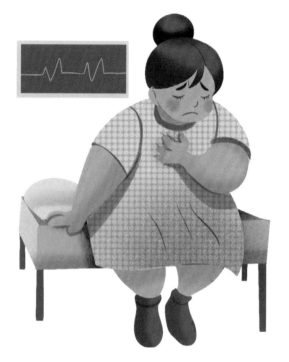

The trends don't look promising. The percentage of students who eat vegetables three or more times a day has declined over the past ten years from 10.1 percent in 2009 to 9.4 percent in 2019.[23] Poor nutrition is another factor contributing to excess weight.

The artists picture Oklahomans rising to the challenge to improve their health and reverse course on obesity's impacts of shortening the length and quality of their lives.

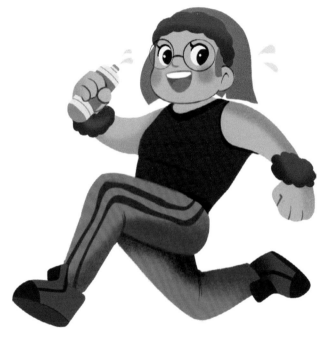

The girl who was previously inactive is energized by running and drinking water to improve her health. The artists also show the power of relationships as individuals with varying levels of fitness work out at their own pace in an encouraging environment. The artists understand issues such as obesity benefit from open discussion and a supportive community of family, friends, and people we admire.

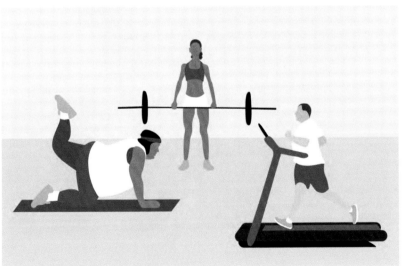

OBESITY

The artists first portray a healthy heart, now whole and filled with luscious fruits and vegetables. Next, the once despondent woman has changed the way she eats and is enjoying healthy food, glowing with optimism, and no longer worrying about chest pains. She now has access to healthier affordable food in her local supermarket.

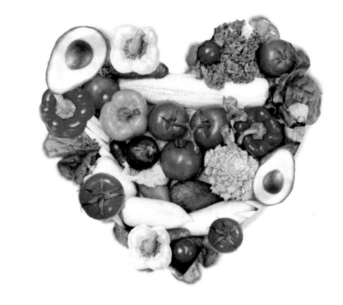

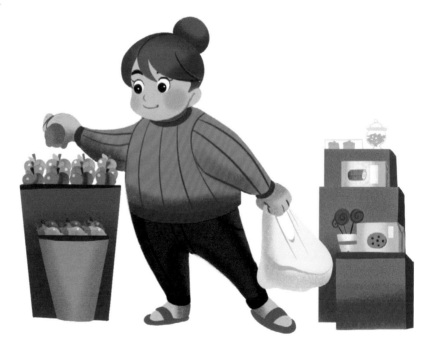

You may not know this yet, but you have the ability to reinvent yourself, endlessly. That's your beauty.[24]

~ LIDIA YUCKNAVICH
AMERICAN AUTHOR, TEACHER AND EDITOR

Prison is a second-by-second assault on the soul, a day-to-day degradation of the self, an oppressive steel and brick umbrella that transforms seconds into hours and hours into days.[1]

~ MUMIA ABU JAMAL

INCARCERATION

T he United States has less than 5 percent of the world's population and nearly 20 percent of its prisoners.[2] While the national incarceration rate is 419 persons per 100,000 of the population, Oklahoma incarcerates people at a significantly higher rate: 639 per 100,000, earning it the second highest ranking in the nation.[3] In 2015, 75 percent of Oklahomans admitted to prison were incarcerated for non-violent crimes, with long sentences given to many of these individuals.[4]

The effects of incarceration on health can be lifelong; individuals with a history of imprisonment have poorer physical and mental health.[5] [6] Imprisonment comes with a high price tag: For fiscal year (FY) 2015, locking up people in Oklahoma was 13 times more expensive than probation or parole supervision.[7]

To present the consequences and dilemmas that accompany such high incarceration rates, the artists create vivid images to illustrate the challenges faced by so many Oklahomans when they enter the prison system.

In 2015, 75 percent of Oklahomans admitted to prison were incarcerated for non-violent crimes. Locking up people in Oklahoma is 13 times more expensive than probation or parole supervision.

Witness the despair of an incarcerated single mother visiting with her children, one of the majority of women imprisoned in Oklahoma for non-violent often drug-related crimes. Her tears illustrate the heartbreaking reality of being separated from her children and her worries about the negative consequences for them that could lead to poor health throughout their lives.[8] [9]

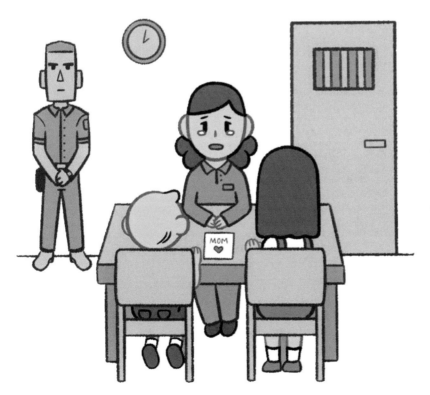

Did you know that Oklahoma has the highest female imprisonment rate in the nation, more than twice as high as the national average?

In an optimistic departure from the reality of today, artists show us a future with a variety of alternatives to prison. At the same time, they recognize the need to tackle core issues such as trauma, poverty and systemic racism that result in excessive imprisonment for minorities. Their ideas express the possibility of better health and cost savings for Oklahomans in the years to come.

In this collection of illustrations, photos and graphics, the artists imagine a way forward that could lead to better lives for many Oklahomans. They recognize Oklahoma needs to address the range of factors that lead to incarceration such as poor education and housing, poverty, lack of community development, insufficient employment preparation tied to future workforce demands, and the need for improved family engagement.[10] The students understand treatment for addiction, substance abuse, and mental health problems is far more effective and less expensive than incarceration. All of these needs play a role in addressing the differences that exist in the excessive numbers of incarcerated people of color.

Oklahoma strategies are recommended that build on these artists' visions such as proven prison diversion programs such as Women in Recovery in Tulsa and REMERGE in Oklahoma City. Given recent statutory changes which modified certain felony offenses to misdemeanors, gatekeepers for mental health and drug courts, including those at a municipal level, should be authorized to determine eligibility of persons suitable for these services. These programs are far less expensive than the $19,000 per prisoner Oklahoma spends annually.[11] [12] Other potential strategies include finding alternate funding for the court system rather than fees and fines which exacerbate factors contributing to poverty such as overwhelming debt. Such funding changes benefit groups most affected: poor people, minorities and those with mental health conditions. [13] [14] [15] [16] County governments would see savings by not detaining non-violent offenders prior to trials.[17] These kinds of strategies, along with others, can help Oklahoma reduce its incarceration rate to the national average, and potentially save more than $160 million annually.[18]

More importantly, improvements in all these areas advance the quality of life, health and well-being of individuals, families, and communities in Oklahoma. In a profound way these strategies will significantly move our state forward.

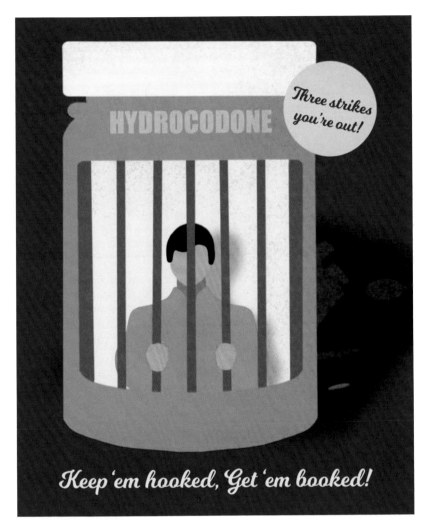

Before recent legislative reforms, the third drug offense in Oklahoma could lead to life imprisonment, an example of severe sentence enhancements often seen for nonviolent crimes. In this way, prisons became the treatment setting of last resort. At this time, a shortage of treatment facilities magnifies this problem.

The artists use the image of "sardines in a can" to reflect on Oklahoma's overcrowded prison system. Outstretched hands may symbolize desperation, a cry for help, a yearning to be treated humanely, all conditions that can be a consequence of Oklahoma's high incarceration rates.

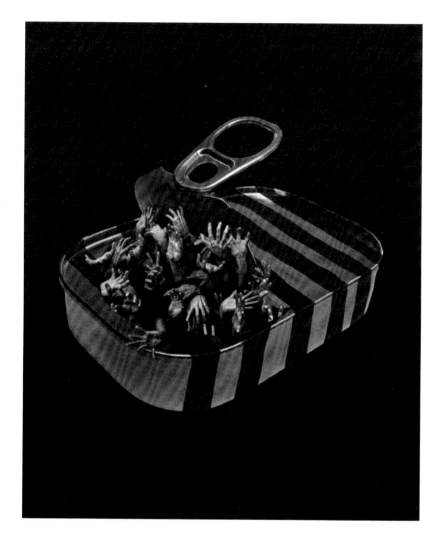

In Oklahoma, Black or African Americans are imprisoned at a rate 4.5 times higher than whites; it is a reminder of racism and stereotypes, punitive prison policies and communities that are not prospering.[19]

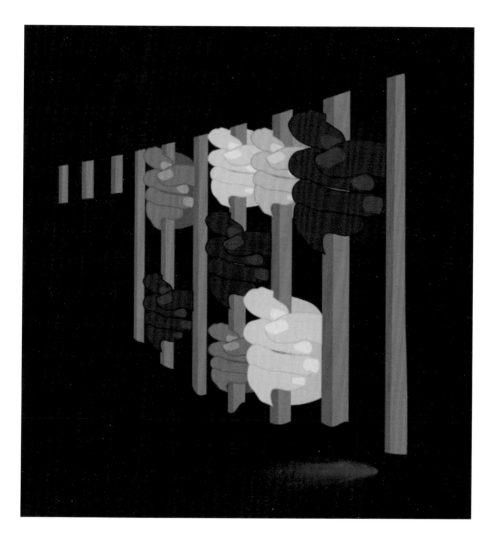

In this illustration, the artists use prison bars in the shape of an Oklahoma map as a symbol of our widespread incarceration rates. Hands clutching bars mirror the unequal racial representation of Oklahoma's prison population.

*"I'm Jennie.
I served ten years
behind bars for
having marijuana."*

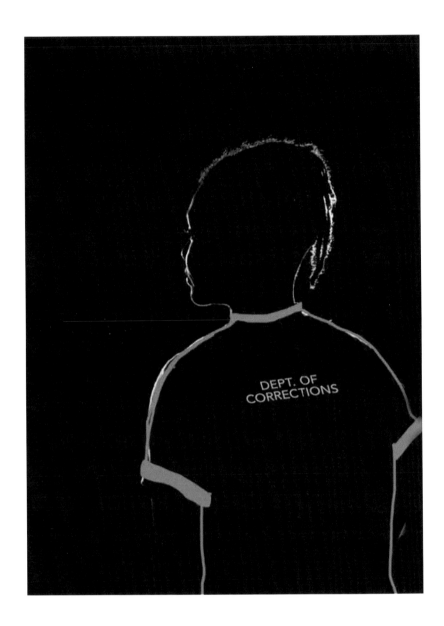

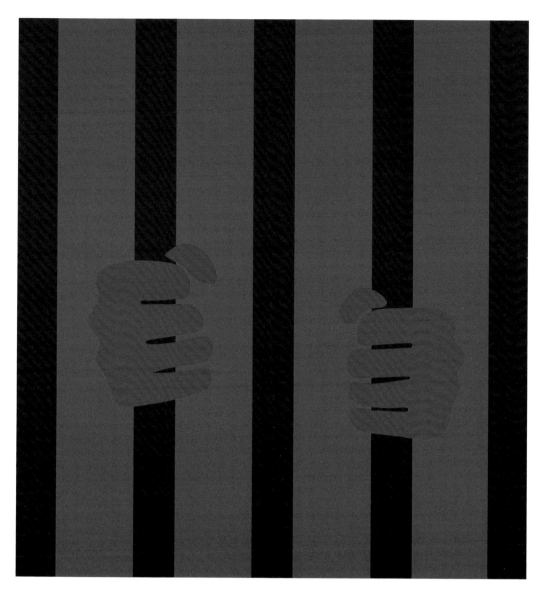

The artists choose stark black bars and a grey background
to illustrate the bleak reality of prison. Red hands clutch
the bars, faceless and without bodily form, perhaps
characterizing the dehumanizing prison experience where
incarceration can result in violence, trauma, diseases, and
chronic stress.[20]

In an optimistic departure from the reality of today, artists show us a future with a variety of alternatives to prison. At the same time, they recognize the need to tackle core issues such as trauma, poverty and systemic racism that result in excessive imprisonment for minorities. Their ideas express the possibility of better health and cost savings for Oklahomans in the years to come.

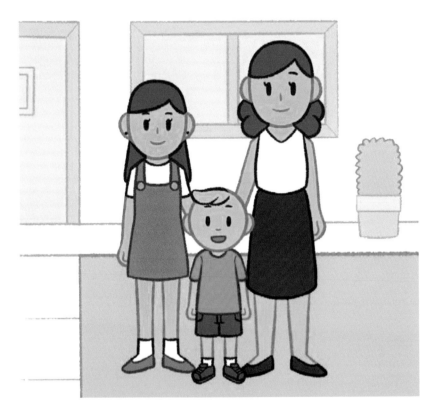

The artists envision this mother participating in alternative preventive programs available in Oklahoma that allow her to stay at home with her children and avoid prison. Her facial expression conveys the joy of the moment, and perhaps her optimism about the employment training she received and the job she was able to obtain as a result. Her children look happy too, spared from the consequences of long-term separation from their mother.[21]

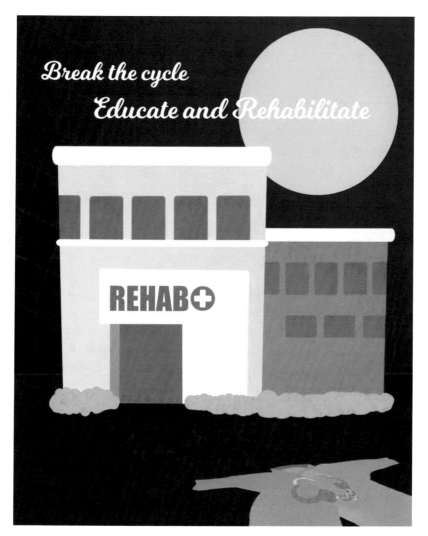

Break the cycle
Educate and Rehabilitate

REHAB✚

Oklahoma now recognizes the positive impact of addressing substance abuse and addiction as early as possible, long before these conditions progress to the point where involvement with the criminal justice system is more likely. The artists' illustration of a treatment center with a bright sun and broken shackles symbolizes the positive future that is possible.

Studies show comprehensive treatment for those suffering from addiction early on is more effective and much less costly than imprisonment. Addressing the shortage of treatment facilities is critical to achieving this goal.

INCARCERATION

*The artists see
education, training,
and employment
opportunities for
those who need
such services to
help prevent crime
in disadvantaged
communities. Perhaps,
as the men work,
looking at a bright
sky, they are grateful
for a system that
helped them achieve
their potential and
avoid prison. All the
better that it saves
vital state funds that
can be used to help
other communities.*

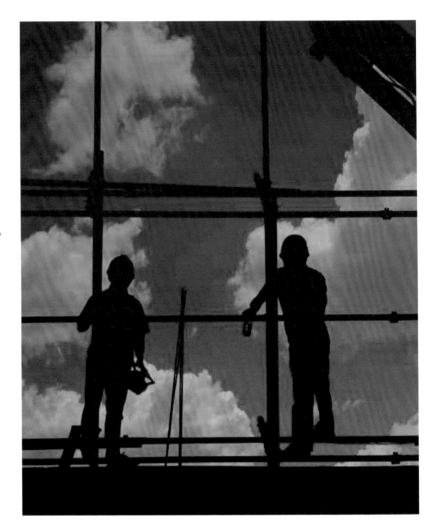

INCARCERATION

60

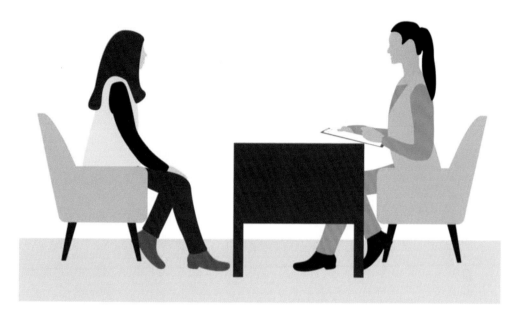

These artists picture a second chance through employment training for a woman who faced imprisonment. Through her training, she learned how to write a resume and develop interview skills for prospective jobs. She looks confident. She's ready to embrace her new job and an optimistic future.

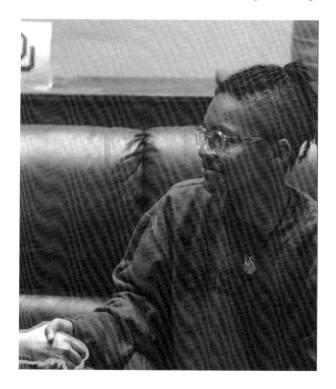

"I'm Jennie. My employer was empathetic and now I get to restart my life."

INCARCERATION

61

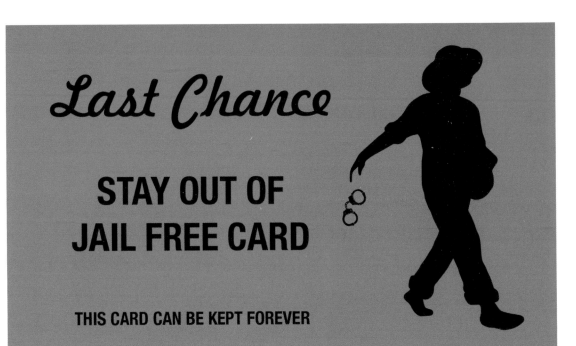

Last Chance

**STAY OUT OF
JAIL FREE CARD**

THIS CARD CAN BE KEPT FOREVER

The artists imagine a future where staying out of jail is an opportunity to help someone who made a mistake create a better future. Handcuffs fall to the ground as a person moves away from a life of crime and instead turns toward living with purpose and direction.

INCARCERATION

As I walked out the door toward my freedom, I knew that if I did not leave all the anger, hatred and bitterness behind that I would still be in prison.[22]

~ NELSON MANDELA
PRESIDENT OF SOUTH AFRICA
FROM 1994 TO 1999

It's hard to raise a child when you are still a child.[1]

ANONYMOUS

TEEN BIRTH RATE

This is the underlying pressure confronting every teen parent. Just as they are in the midst of their own development, teens are thrust into having the responsibility of caring for one so tiny and vulnerable. That is why it is heartening to report that teen pregnancy rates have reached all-time lows in the nation and state. Teens abstaining from sex as well as effective use of birth control have contributed to these reductions.[2] Yet while all of this is good news, Oklahoma's teen birth rate of 10.6 births per 1,000 females aged 15–17 years of age is still higher than the national average of 7.2. For 2017, Oklahoma scored an F on the *State of the State's Health* Report.[3][4][5]

The artists illustrate, through a collage of pictures, the struggles teenage girls face upon realizing they are pregnant. Here are their stories.

Oklahoma's teen birth rate scored an F on the State of the State's Health *report card.*

This image of educational material almost entirely redacted lets us know there is important information that is not seen when educating our youth about responsible sexual behavior. It is this very lack of knowledge that contributes to Oklahoma's high teen birth rate.. A fuller, more open conversation can change the direction of children having babies.

Contraction ▮▮▮▮▮▮▮▮▮▮▮▮▮▮▮▮ Complete abstinence ▮▮▮▮▮▮▮▮▮▮▮▮▮▮▮ effective method ▮▮▮▮▮▮▮▮▮▮▮▮▮ effective ▮▮▮▮ ▮▮▮▮▮▮▮▮▮▮▮▮▮ prevents sperm form reaching the egg, is very reliable. ▮▮▮▮▮▮▮▮▮▮▮▮▮ ▮▮▮▮▮▮▮▮▮▮▮▮▮▮▮▮▮▮▮▮▮▮ ▮▮▮▮▮▮▮ vasectomy, ▮▮▮▮▮▮▮▮▮▮▮▮ ▮▮▮▮▮▮▮▮▮▮▮▮▮▮▮▮▮▮▮▮▮▮ ▮▮▮▮▮▮▮▮▮▮▮▮▮▮▮▮▮▮▮▮▮▮ ▮▮▮▮▮▮▮▮▮▮▮▮▮▮▮▮▮▮▮▮▮▮

The effectiveness of other methods of contraception ▮▮▮▮ ▮▮▮▮▮▮▮▮▮▮ abstinence, ▮▮▮▮▮▮ ▮▮▮▮▮▮▮▮▮ natural family planning, ▮▮▮ refraining from intercourse ▮▮▮▮▮▮▮▮▮▮ ▮▮▮▮▮▮▮▮▮▮▮▮▮▮▮▮▮▮▮▮▮▮ ▮▮▮▮▮▮▮▮▮▮▮▮▮▮▮▮▮▮▮▮▮▮ ▮▮▮▮▮▮▮▮▮▮▮▮▮▮▮▮▮▮▮▮▮▮ ▮▮▮▮▮▮▮▮▮▮▮▮▮▮▮▮▮▮▮▮▮▮ ▮▮▮▮▮▮▮▮▮▮▮▮▮▮▮▮▮▮▮

LET'S TALK ＿＿＿＿＿＿＿＿＿＿＿＿ .

These artists are telling us that education is a key component to reduce teen pregnancy in our state. Parents and other trusted adults play an important role in helping teens make healthy choices about relationships, sex and birth control. Comprehensive sex education, including but not limited to abstinence, needs to take place at our schools and at safe places where youth meet. Additionally, there needs to be easy access to contraceptive and reproductive health services.[6] For at-risk or poor students, youth development programs can keep teens in schools, provide after-school activities and teach life skills, all ways to broaden available options for these young adults.[7] Local initiatives, especially in disadvantaged communities where there are high teenage pregnancy rates, are important to reduce disparities where there are racial, ethnic and geographic differences. Local projects create partnerships between key organizations to offer services, educate the public on 'what works', and create awareness about the relationship between teen pregnancy and conditions in their communities.[8 9 10 11 12 13 14 15]

It will take a combination of changes by individuals, families and communities to achieve lasting reductions in teenage pregnancy rates. All of these strategies will improve individual and collective health.

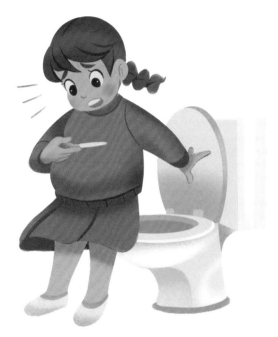

Notice the look of surprise and concern on these teenagers' faces. Their situation seems bleak since they just learned they are pregnant. Now images of graduation hang in the shadows. The hopes they once held for a better future now seem like impossible dreams to achieve. They both wish they had been better informed and learned how to protect themselves.

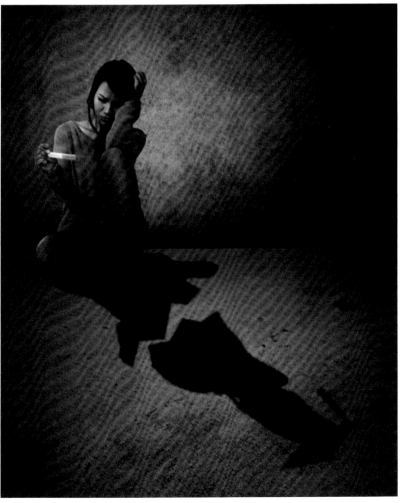

TEEN BIRTH RATE

67

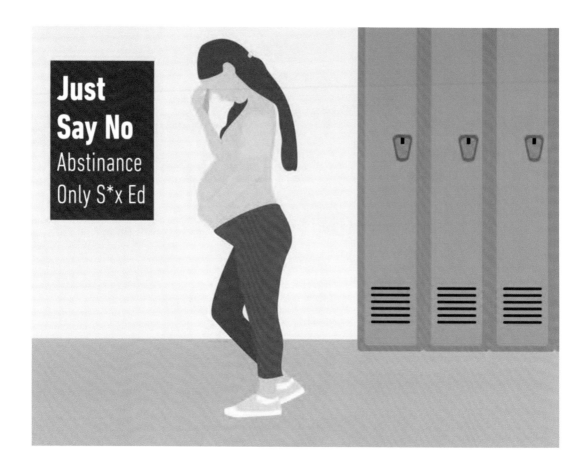

The artist expresses the limitation of "just say no." Another pregnant teenager in our schools. This approach eliminates consideration of options important in a world where many teenagers are sexually active. In fact, 43 percent of high school youth in Oklahoma report having had sex.[16] [17] This teenager looks trapped, now left to wonder how to manage motherhood at such a young age.

Medical and financial support during pregnancy and the first year of a baby's life is $16,000 per teen birth.[18] Is there a better way to educate and inform our teens about responsible sexual behavior and the obligations that come with parenthood?

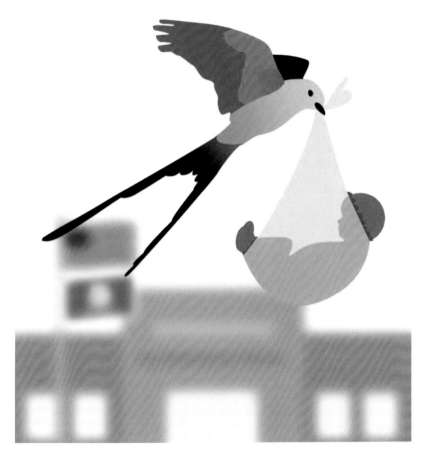

This scissortail is a reminder of the consequences driving Oklahoma's teen birth rate. This happens when there are limited conversations between youth, their families and staff at their local schools. It is as if babies are dropping into our communities.

Teen pregnancies carry medical risks, with these girls having a greater chance of high blood pressure, anemia, premature births, low birthweight babies and postpartum depression.[19] Pregnancy and birth are significant contributors to high school dropout rates among girls. The children of teenage mothers are also more likely to drop out of high school, have more health problems, be incarcerated at some time during adolescence, give birth as a teenager, and face unemployment as a young adult. Lower education and income levels can also contribute to high teenage pregnancy rates.[20]

TEEN BIRTH RATE

These students seem despondent, weighed down by the burden of having to care for their infants. They wanted to fit in so they went along with the crowd and now find themselves saddled with newborn babies. This just adds to their worries, a consequence they will live with day and night.

"I'm Amy. I got pregnant before I could even think about college."

TEEN BIRTH RATE

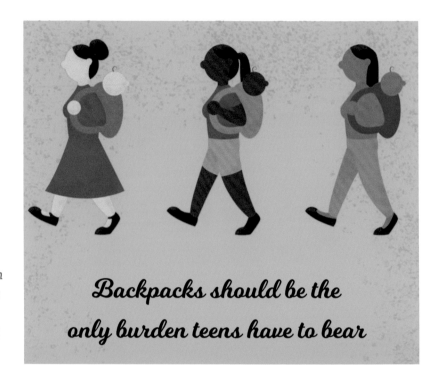

Backpacks should be the only burden teens have to bear

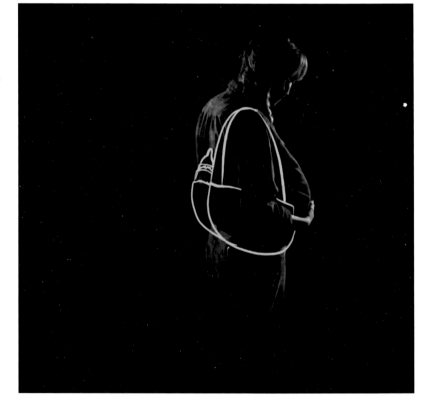

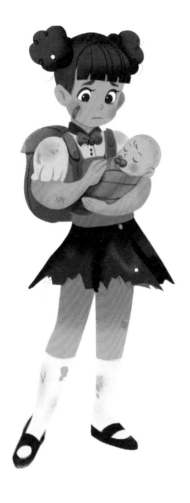

This girl seems sad since she now knows that having a baby may mean a life of hardship. It is hard to stay in school and work to make ends meet. Does this teen wish she would have waited now that she is raising the baby by herself?

Two-thirds of teen mothers who move out of their family home live in poverty, and a similar share receive public benefits in the first year of their child's life.[21]

TEEN BIRTH RATE

The artists provide needed consistent messaging to frame their solutions. They strongly declare that a comprehensive sex education curriculum is the answer to give teens, both male and female, the tools and knowledge needed to prevent teen pregnancy. Learning has to include effective use of contraceptives. Education and birth control need to be in locations that are convenient and safe.

Now the students are getting the information they need. There are conversations with both boys and girls since both groups know they need to be responsible for their actions. All this information provides answers to formerly unspoken questions.

Contraception is the deliberate prevention of pregnancy. Complete abstinence (avoiding intercourse) is the only totally effective method of birth control, but other methods are effective to varying degrees. Sterilization, surgery that prevents sperm form reaching the egg, is very reliable. A woman may have a **tubal ligation** ("having her tubes tied"), in which a doctor removes a short section from each oviduct, often tying (ligating) the remaining ends. A man may undergo a **vasectomy**, in which a doctor cuts a section out of each vas deferens to prevent sperm from reaching the uterus. Both forms of sterilization are relatively safe and free from side effects. Sterilization procedures are generally considerd permanent, but sometimes can be surgically reversed. Surgical reversals of tubal ligations or vasectomies are becoming increasingly successful, but these major surgeries carry some risk.

The effectiveness of other methods of contraception depends on how they are used. Temporary abstinence, also called the **rhythm method** or **natural family planning**, depends on the refraining from intercourse during the days around ovulation, when fertilization's most likely. In theory, the time of ovulation can be determined by monitoring changes in body temperature and the composition of cervical mucus, but careful monitoring and record keeping are required. Additionally, the length of the reproductive cycle can vary from month to month, and sperm can survive for 3–5 days within the females reproductive track making family planning quite unreliable in actual practice. Withdrawal of the penis from the vigina before ejaculation is also ineffective because the sperm may rereleased before climax.

LET'S TALK TEEN PREGNANCY.

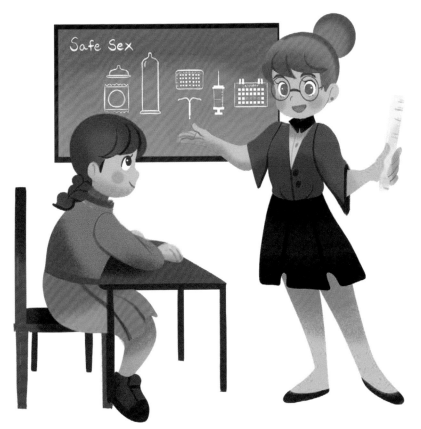

This teen is now taught all she needs to know because of her comprehensive sexual education classes. She did not realize there was so much to learn. Now she can resist any peer pressure and delay having sex until she is ready. At that time, she will know how to protect herself with the best available contraceptives.

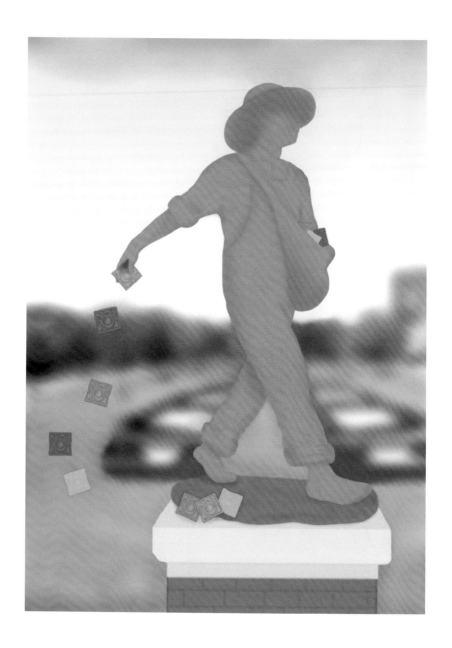

TEEN BIRTH RATE

74

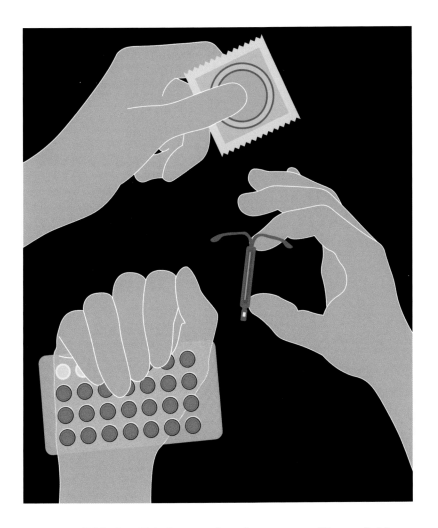

Now, all kinds of birth control options are readily available for when teens choose to become sexually active. Teens are getting good information on how to take charge of their own behavior. They know it is a shared responsibility.

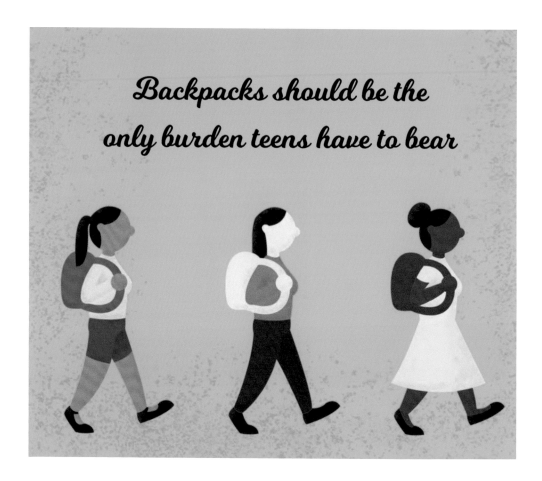

Backpacks should be the only burden teens have to bear

These girls are glad they did not respond to peer pressure from their friends to have sex before they were ready. They know school is hard enough and they are grateful they can concentrate on their studies full time. By delaying sex, these youth will not contribute to another generation of teen births. It is like you can see them smiling, with a bounce in their steps as they see a sure path forward.

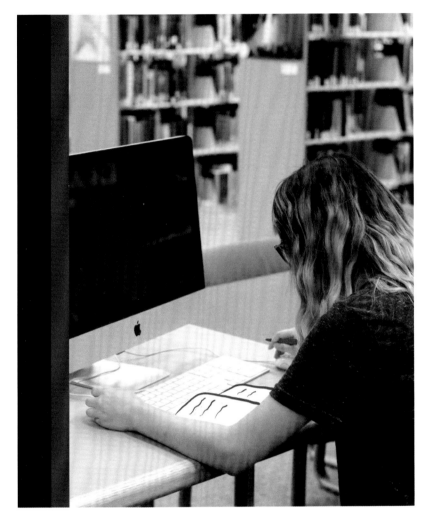

"I'm Amy. Now I'm working to get my GED."

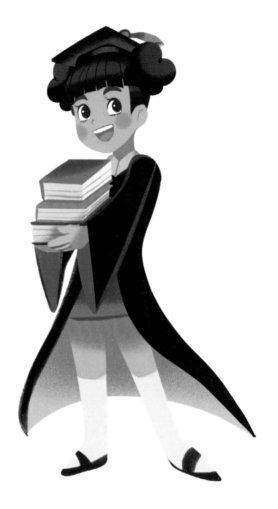

This teen is so glad she waited to have a baby. Now she is graduating with honors and imagines a world full of possibilities once she completes her college degree. This teen knows she wants to be a parent in the future. She looks forward to having a baby once she is able to support herself and meet the responsibilities of being a parent.

Reducing teen pregnancy and birth is one of the most effective ways of reducing child poverty in the country.[22]

~ JORDAN BROWN

You cannot solve the teen pregnancy problem once and for all. It requires ongoing effort and investment to make sure every new generation is educated and has access to services.[23]

~ BOSTON CHILDREN'S HOSPITAL

CONDITIONS AFFECTING OUR HEALTH

Poverty is a constant state of insecurity. Poverty is choosing between food and electricity. Poverty is exhaustion, in every way. Poverty is being hungry.[1]

~ SHAUNTA GRIMES

POVERTY

Poverty is a balancing act. It is choosing among necessities with little or no room to maneuver. At its core, poverty is when people do not have enough money to meet basic needs such as food, clothing and shelter.[2] In 2019 Oklahoma's poverty rate was 15.2 percent, almost 2.9 percentage points higher than the national rate of 12.3 percent.[3] Oklahoma ranks as the 9th worst state in the nation where 21.7 percent of our children live in poverty.[4] More than 1 in 10 Oklahoma children live in what is called "concentrated poverty"— neighborhoods where 30 percent or more of the population lives below the federal poverty line.[5][6][7] The long-term results of these conditions: poor people are more likely to live less healthy, shorter lives.[8][9][10]

Oklahoma ranks as the 9th worst state in the nation for childhood poverty.

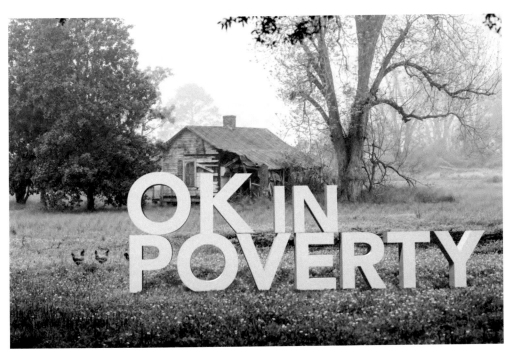

Poverty permeates too many of our rural communities as well as our urban centers. Too many Oklahomans are forced to live in unsightly and dilapidated dwellings, unable to afford anything better. Is it really okay for someone to live in a rundown, unsafe house with broken windows, peeling paint and overgrown trees? Some towns and cities in Oklahoma are dotted with these structures that present a threat to the health and well-being of people and the overall community.

Poor people living in cities fare no better. The artists imagine, for this man, that his home is a campsite, his cardboard sign a sad announcement of his plight. They see that he exists in daily adversity against a landscape of boarded-up structures, from meal to meal, in unending mobile misery, with danger lurking at every corner. Even as he sleeps, you can see his distress as he desperately clutches his beleaguered face for self-comfort and protection.

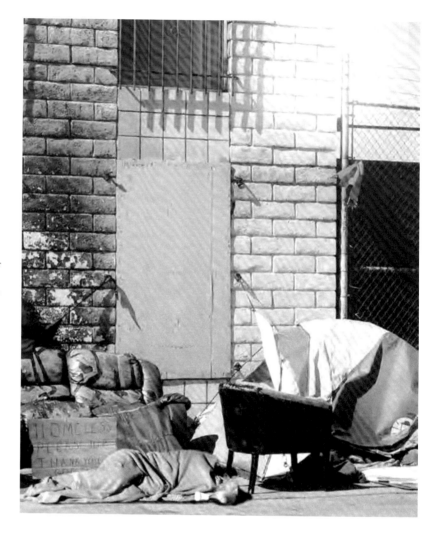

The artists are showing us the importance education plays in escaping poverty. Those with more education have higher incomes which is a strong predictor of health. Better education and strong community resources require structural changes in disadvantaged communities to achieve a more level playing field with equal opportunities for everyone.

The artists confirm how education is a critical piece in eliminating poverty. It is the way to end the financial insecurity resulting from joblessness or low-wage jobs, unaffordable housing, lack of preventive care and untreated chronic medical conditions.[11]

Learning should continue over one's lifespan, starting with quality early childhood programs and extending through post-graduate degrees. We know it will take more than a high school diploma to meet future workforce needs. A partnership between higher education and business is necessary to couple educational achievement with job skills that help individuals advance and change careers over a lifetime.[12] For those starting off, work should result in families being able to meet basic needs. Raising the minimum wage and returning the refundability of the state's earned income tax credit, along with increasing its amount, would be good first steps to help working adults support their families.[13]

Affordable health care is crucial. It will provide individuals with more disposable income and prevent delays in seeking needed medical care which can be more costly in the future. Reducing the number of uninsured in our state took a giant step forward when Oklahomans approved the state initiative to expand Medicaid. However, more funding is needed to serve individuals not covered by the expansion and for treatment services for physical, mental and substance abuse problems, especially in areas where low-income families reside.

The artists illustrate, in a moving manner, the consequences of unstable housing. They know that safe, secure shelter is a needed component to sustain health, free of the worries of crime and environmental harm.[14]

Tackling poverty is key to improving the quality of life for all Oklahomans and producing savings in what we spend for social services, medical care and law enforcement to name a few. Our children deserve to live in communities where they can learn, play, and grow.[15] Reducing poverty will require bold actions through long-term engagement between local and state leaders in education, workforce, health, human service and housing sectors. Just as it took courage and determination to garner support for a federal highway system, let's vow to do "what it takes" to give future generations of Oklahomans the ability to live better than those who came before them.

*"I'm Amelia.
I was so hungry every
night but could not
afford more."*

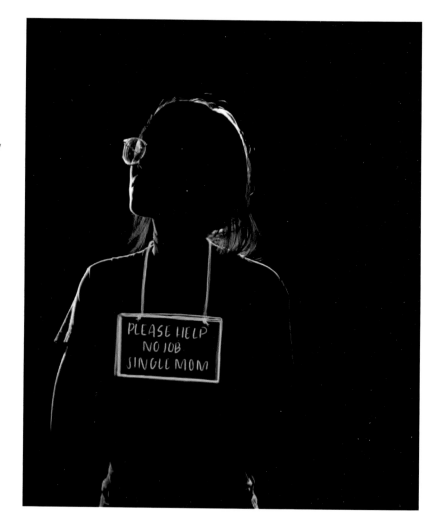

*Black or African Americans are six times and Latinos four
times more likely to live in communities with concentrated
poverty.[16] For them and their families, they live in constant
stress with few options for well-paying jobs, adequate
housing and safe neighborhoods.[17] Children in poverty are
at risk for a host of issues such as hunger, poor health,
and academic failure.[18] [19]*

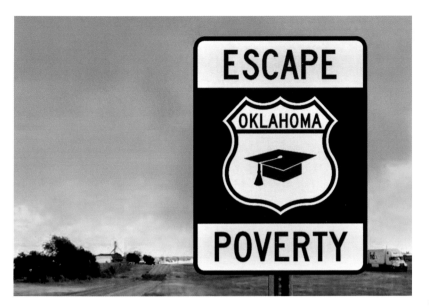

The artists provide us with a sign offering a way forward for Oklahoma's future. It expresses the same optimistic vision that created Route 66 in the early 20th century, when a national highway was a symbol of growth, change and progress for the whole nation. This new sign stands on a horizon amidst a bright Oklahoma landscape teeming with opportunity.

Here we see better possibilities for the homeless in need of services. This welcoming home looks warm and inviting and is called a "Serenity House" by its designers. What a wonderful gift, to have a place offering peace and reflection.

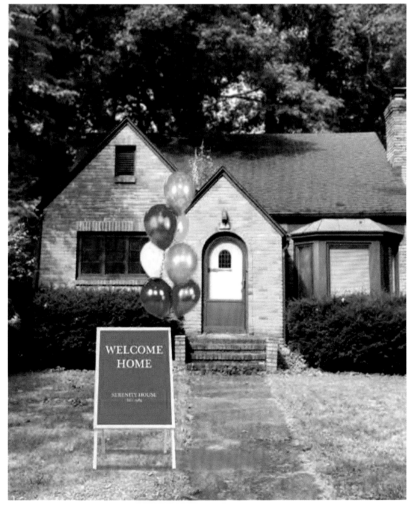

87

*"I'm Amelia.
Now I can feed both
my daughter and me."*

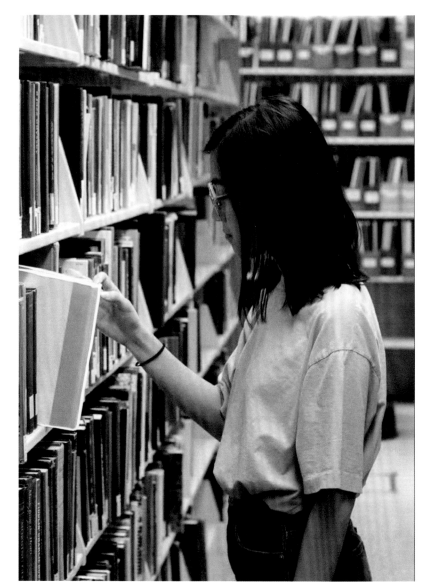

POVERTY

*. . . poverty is not just economic but
defined by way of health and education.*[20]

~ AZIM PREMJI
BUSINESS INVESTOR
ENGINEER AND PHILANTHROPIST

I feel that we cannot educate children who are not healthy, and we can't keep them healthy if they are not educated. There has to be a marriage between health and education. ...[1]

~ JOCELYN ELDERS
FORMER SURGEON GENERAL
OF THE UNITED STATES

EDUCATION

American businesses need an educated workforce to compete with other countries for the specialized occupations that exist now and in the future.[2] Increased education, for example four years of college, is associated with increased life expectancy and improved health. For 2018, Oklahoma's overall high school graduation rate of 82 percent was lower than the national average by 3 percent with worse results for low-income households, Blacks, American Indians, Hispanics and students with disabilities.[3][4][5]

Oklahoma ranks 43rd in the nation in PreK –12 education and 39th overall.[6]

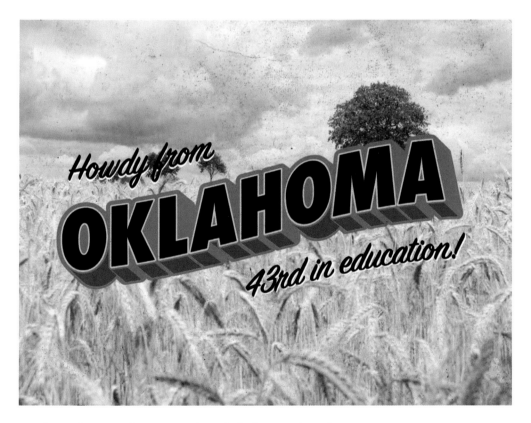

The artists are demonstrating their frustration about Oklahoma's national ranking in education. We see an iconic Oklahoma image exposing our poor outcomes. Things have to change so that the beauty of the waving wheat is matched by the pride we have in our educational excellence. For these artists, our welcoming "howdy" needs to meet the moment of what Oklahoma offers: great education, good jobs, and a place that families are proud to call their home.

91

In 2019, the percent of Oklahomans age 25 and over with a bachelor's degree or higher was 26.2 percent, lagging behind the national rate at 33.1 percent.[7] A middle path between a high school diploma and a bachelor's degree—receiving credentials, certifications or associate's degrees—shows that 40% of Oklahomans have these types of accreditations with a goal to reach 70% by 2025.[8][9]

The artists through these pictures demonstrate the shortcomings of low educational achievement in the state. The students also remind us that educational accomplishments do not exist in isolation; they are part of the larger environment in which children and youth live.

Learning must begin early. The state needs to expand the number of high quality early childhood programs for young children in both urban and rural settings to lay down a solid foundation of intellectual and social development.[10][11] As children progress, we now know what it takes for students to successfully complete high school: regular attendance, good grades and enrollment in rigorous courses that prepare them for college.[12] To achieve this, Oklahoma will need to invest more in supports for at-risk students as well as funding increases to address differences between low and high poverty school districts.[13] For minority and low-income students, a positive engaged and respectful school culture, that attends to school safety and students' social and emotional learning, is critical to increase the quality of their education.[14][15][16]

School-based health-care centers (SBHC) are a cost effective way to help with many of the stresses faced by students and their families. SBHC's are ideal settings to address the health and social barriers to educational success through physical and mental health care and educational programming.[17]

There are many strategies available to increase college completion rates: additional high school funding for college credit courses, easier transfer of college credits, expansion of online education and more partnerships between higher education and business to name a few.[18]

To improve health, we need policies that set kids up for success in education and life. While medical care is important, education, jobs and economic growth are the best ways to improve health outcomes and reduce costs, especially in those communities with the greatest needs.[19] Education and health go hand in hand. These individual, community and state strategies recognize the connection between them.[20]

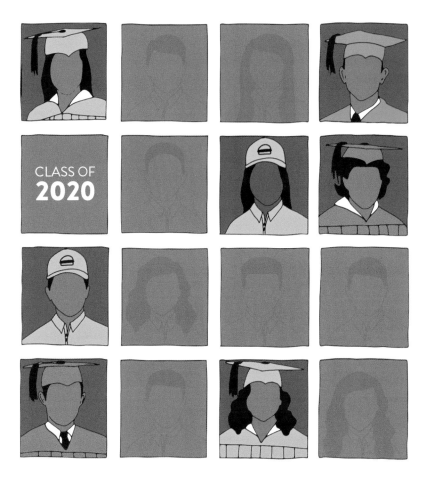

CLASS OF
2020

The artists seem to be asking why so many students are missing? What happened to them? They worry that dropping out will result in a future of low-wage jobs. Dropping out is a trap in which students' destinies are typically a lifetime of poverty and poor health.

Educational attainment is linked to better health. Better educated Americans are more likely to have higher incomes with health insurance coverage, live in better neighborhoods, adopt healthier behaviors and experience less stress for themselves and their families. The results for these individuals are lower medical costs and longer and better health throughout their lives.[21] [22] Finding ways to increase the number of Oklahomans who improve their educational status could get us to a future where Oklahomans are both well-off and well![23]

EDUCATION

We see an empty, barren classroom. Everything is outdated: a chalkboard, old desks and pads of paper and pencils. The artists wonder about the level of student support, imagining substitute teachers as a regular occurrence. Students in this classroom don't have anything they need to compete in today's computer-centered high-tech world. It puts them at a disadvantage when they apply for college.

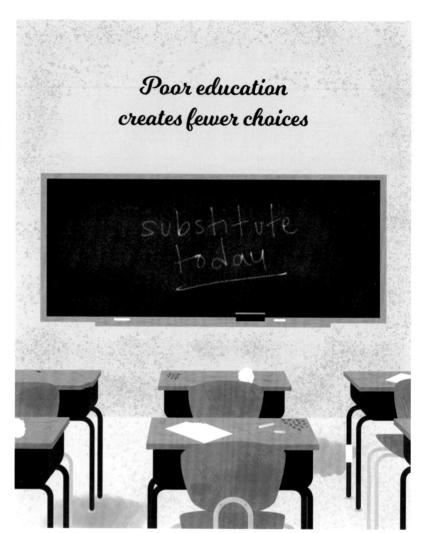

Poor education creates fewer choices

With over 50 percent of Oklahoman students living in poor families, many children and youth find themselves stuck in low performing schools, reflecting the challenges their communities have in adapting to economic and social changes in our society.[24]

Yet, if Oklahoma adopts reforms to strengthen the state's overall educational system, our artists can imagine a future with increased prosperity and well-being for its residents. The artists portray a world full of possibilities because of strong levels of educational achievement.

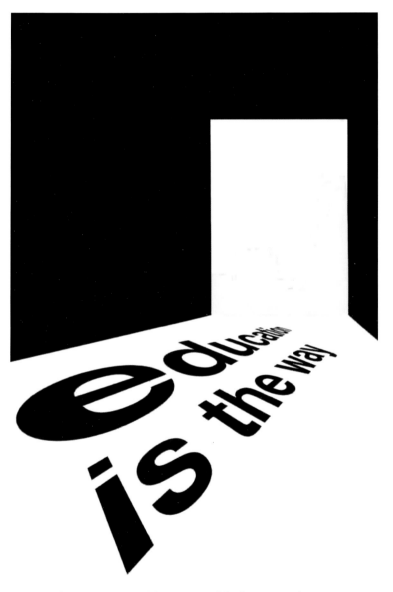

The artists see a bright and optimistic future with education paving the way. Big letters at the top illustrate how important it is for children to get a strong educational foundation early in their lives. Each letter is a progression from kindergarten through high school, leading to a college diploma hanging from an office wall.

Improving educational levels would also save the state money. Did you know Oklahoma could save over $50 million in Medicaid costs if the state reduced the percentage of youth not completing high school by 50 percent?[25]

The artists show us a class full of happy, hopeful students getting their diplomas. This is what a 100 percent high school graduation rate looks like. What are their dreams? Are they on to college for additional degrees? Will they be getting skills that allow them to be financially secure? They have prepared themselves for a better future.

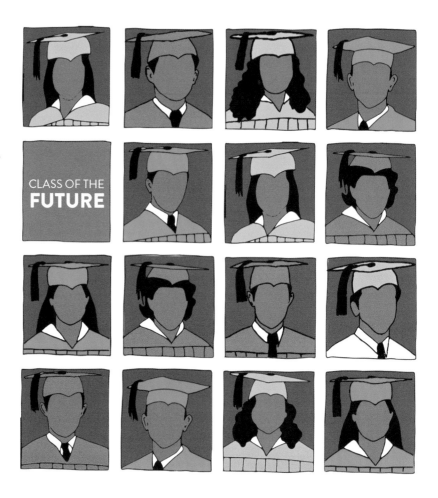

CLASS OF THE
FUTURE

College graduates earn one and a half times more than those only completing high school, 84% more over a lifetime. Better personal health will be a byproduct of these increased earnings, with easier access to health insurance and conditions conducive to a healthier lifestyle.[26] [27] [28]

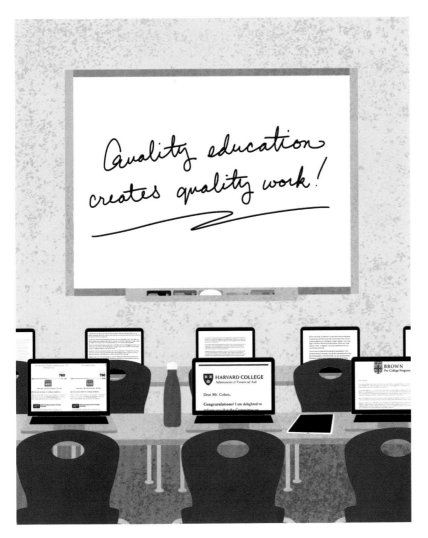

What a difference funding makes! Now there are state of the art classrooms and supplies: a white board, laptops on every desk and modern furniture. The artists imagine amazing, talented teachers supporting high school seniors throughout the school year. Can you guess what happened? Most of these students are graduating with scholarships to wonderful colleges.

You need to make an investment, and the investment is in health and education.[29]

~ BUZZ ALDRIN
AMERICAN ENGINEER
FORMER ASTRONAUT
AND FIGHTER PILOT

It's a disgrace that we have millions of people who are uninsured.[1]

~ COLIN POWELL
FORMER UNITED STATES
SECRETARY OF STATE,
AND RETIRED FOUR-STAR GENERAL U.S. ARMY

UNINSURED

Uninsured people say the high cost of insurance is the primary reason they lack coverage and delay going to the doctor or filling a prescription.[2] [3] [4] Until recently, Oklahoma was one of several states that declined to expand Medicaid, leaving many working adults without health insurance. In 2019, 552,835 Oklahomans did not have health insurance, an increase of over 4,500 individuals from 2018. At 14.3 percent Oklahoma's uninsured rate is the second worst in the nation.[5] [6]

In the images in this chapter, artists portray the challenges facing those without health insurance and access to affordable healthcare.

Oklahoma's uninsured rate, at 14.3 percent, is the second-worst in the nation.

Imagine piles of medical bills and no way to pay them. Those who are uninsured must often choose between paying for food, rent and utilities, or expensive medical bills. Medical debt—a one-night stay in the hospital can cost thousands—and the bills become a financial prison that affects self-esteem and quality of life.

LET'S TALK _____.

In the following images, our artists imagine reversing how things stand. They picture an Oklahoman future where affordable health insurance is available to all.

Increasing the number of people with health insurance is critical to improving health outcomes and decreasing healthcare spending. One way to increase coverage is targeted outreach for enrollment through Medicaid or the ACA healthcare marketplace. Partners exist that already serve many of these potentially eligible individuals— community action agencies, health departments, public schools and cooperative employers in lower-wage industries. Coupling healthcare insurance outreach with enrollment in programs like the Free and Reduced School Meals programs, Women, Infants and Children (WIC) and Supplemental Nutritional Assistance Program (SNAP) further strengthens health outcomes.[7]

Even with Medicaid expansion passed, there are still many hard-working residents in our state where affordable insurance is out of reach. There needs to be continued work to ensure healthcare coverage is available for all Oklahomans. In this way, we can take pride by significantly improving the well-being of thousands of our residents.

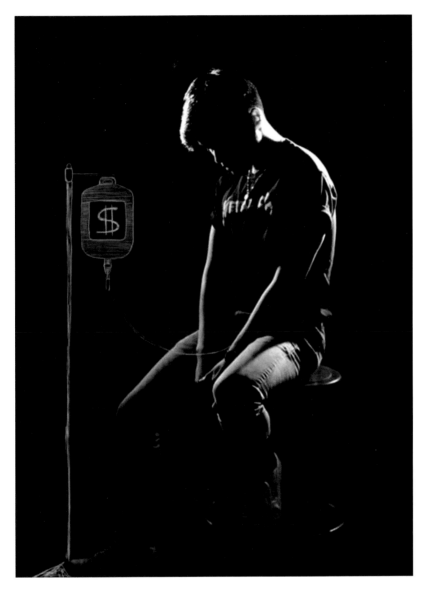

"I'm Patrick. My cancer treatment bills were as overwhelming as my diagnosis."

UNINSURED

101

In this image, the artists portray the outcome of years without healthcare due to a lack of health insurance, a dilemma especially felt by those with chronic medical conditions. The toe tag symbolizes a life devalued for lacking access to affordable healthcare and health insurance. Given significant numbers of Oklahomans facing this predicament, this scenario is tragically far too common.

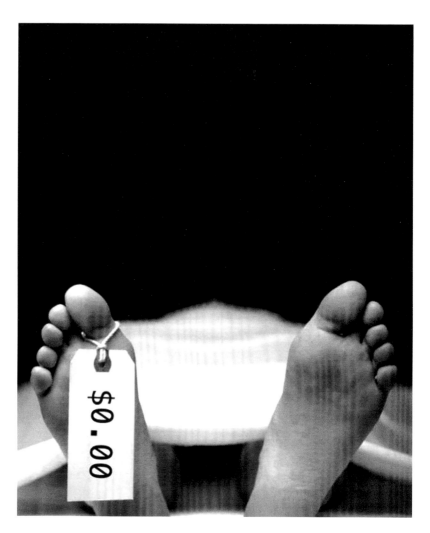

UNINSURED

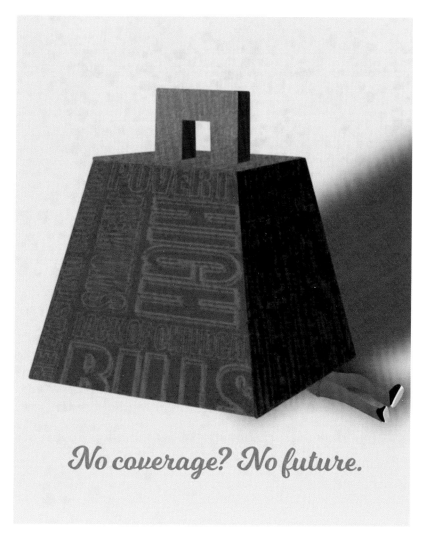

No coverage? No future.

The artists choose a crushing weight atop a person to symbolize living without access to affordable health insurance. Perhaps the artists imagine that with no one to help lift the weight, medical debt is an inevitable and expensive outcome, adding to the anxiety of life without healthcare.

Even with passage of the state question to expand the number of individuals eligible for Medicaid, there will still be many Oklahomans that remain uninsured. Often, they make too much money to qualify for Medicaid but not enough to get good insurance and health care.[8]

UNINSURED

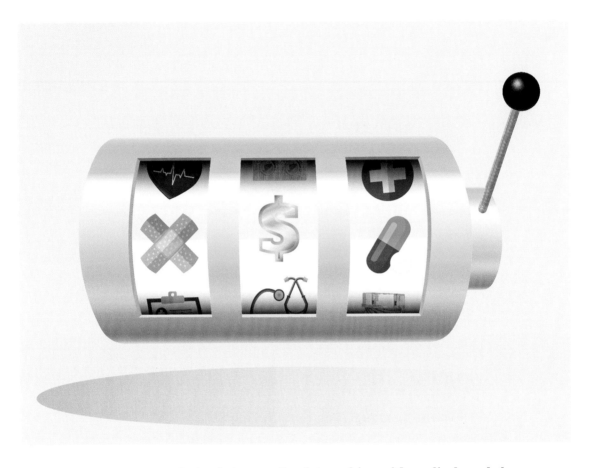

A simple image of a slot machine with medical symbols showcases the artists' keen understanding of life without health insurance. Trapped in a system that gambles with their lives, the uninsured are aware the odds are not in their favor. Oklahoma faces two choices: be proactive and pay upfront with low-cost coverage, or bet with their lives and wait. Waiting means worse outcomes for all. For the uninsured, expensive emergency room visits become primary care, delays in seeing a doctor bloom into expensive hospitalizations, and taxpayers end up footing the tab for the most expensive healthcare system in the world.[9] Last but not least, waiting means a significant percentage of Oklahomans face worse health outcomes and higher rates of death.[10] [11] [12] [13]

In the following images, our artists imagine reversing how things stand. They picture an Oklahoman future where affordable health insurance is available to all.

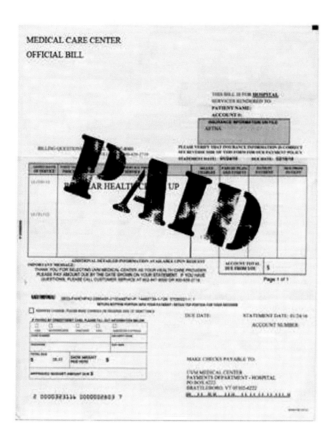

LET'S TALK INSURANCE.

The artists use a "paid" bill to portray how the lives of those formerly uninsured benefit when health insurance pays for medical bills. Now they imagine a sense of relief that comes with regular medical appointments and preventive care to stay healthy.

"I'm Patrick.
Now with health
insurance, I feel like
I can fight the good
fight."

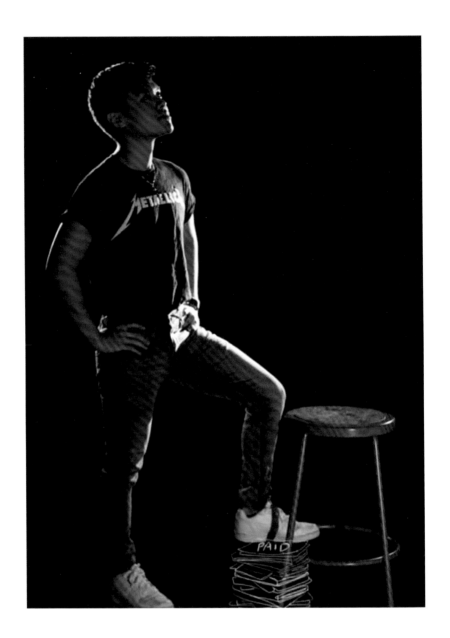

UNINSURED

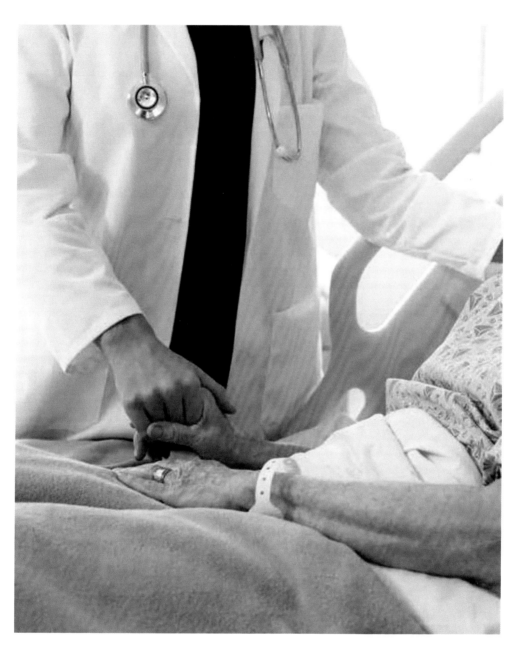

A medical professional holding a patient's hand illustrates an ongoing, supportive patient-doctor relationship. Perhaps the artists desire for all Oklahomans to have access to affordable, quality healthcare paid for by health insurance that covers the treatments people need.

It is easy to imagine artists are expressing the relief Oklahomans feel once legislators pass affordable healthcare for all. Now there are no more burdens of how to afford expensive treatment. The historical weights are gone with Oklahomans no longer worried that medical bills may drive them into extreme medical debt or perhaps even bankruptcy. It is a day to be proud, where Oklahoma is now a leader by providing universal health care.

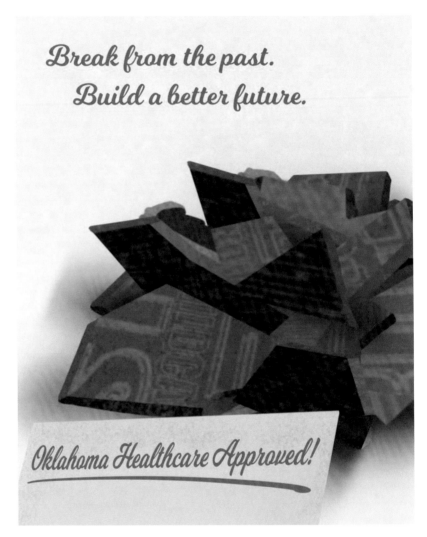

Break from the past.
Build a better future.

Oklahoma Healthcare Approved!

Passage by the voters of the Medicaid expansion is a good first step where it is estimated that enrollment will increase 34 percent; between 178,000 and 233,000 more Oklahomans will be covered by this program. New Medicaid patients will have access to care known to improve health, such as preventative services like tobacco cessation and immunization programs, primary care as well as treatment for mental health and substance abuse disorders. The Medicaid expansion will create jobs; provide savings in other state programs, and is estimated to bring more than $1 billion in tax dollars back to the state of Oklahoma.[14] [15] [16] [17]

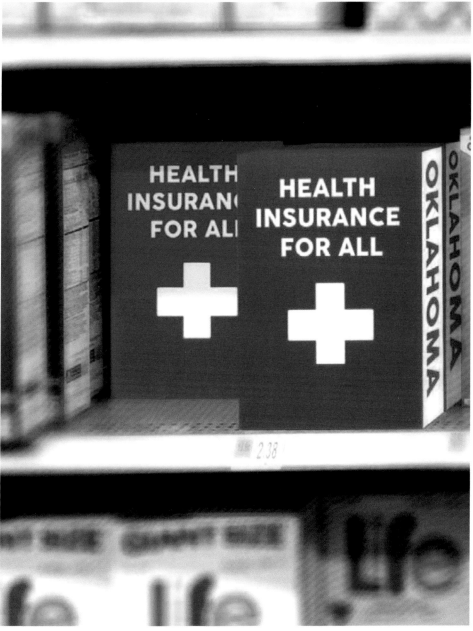

In an Oklahoma with a high quality of life, our artists envision health insurance that is as accessible and plentiful as the cereal options in a grocery store. Are the artists also asking whether we need more health insurance companies? Increased competition could translate into more affordable quality plans with low premiums and deductibles and comprehensive benefits for Oklahomans.[18]

I am a single mother of three kids (one has autism and another has seizures), and have been working on building my own business so that I can be home with my kids. Medicaid coverage is allowing me peace of mind for me and my children.[19]

~ KRISTA
MEDICAID EXPANSION
SUCCESS STORIES

Notes

INTRODUCTION

1   Center for Disease Control and Prevention (CDC), National Centers for Health Statistics, "Infant Mortality by State," Last Reviewed April 24, 2020, https://www.cdc.gov/nchs/pressroom/sosmap/infant__mortality__rates/infant__mortality.htm

2   Center for Disease Control and Prevention, National Center for Health Statistics, "Cancer Mortality by State," Last reviewed April 29, 2020, https://www.cdc.gov/nchs/pressroom/sosmap/cancer__mortality/cancer.htm

3   Oklahoma State Department of Health, *State of the State's Health Report*, accessed June 19, 2020, https://stateofstateshealth.ok.gov/Data/HealthIndicator

4   United Health Foundation, *America's Health Rankings 2019 Annual Report*, 2020 Copyright United Health Foundation, accessed May 31, 2020, https://assets.americashealthrankings.org/app/uploads/ahr__2019annualreport.pdf

5   R.G. Parrish, "Measuring population health outcomes" Prevention of Chronic Disease 2010; Vol 7 No 4: A71, accessed May 31, 2020, https://www.cdc.gov/pcd/issues/2010/jul/10__0005.htm

6   University of Wisconsin, Population Health Institute, School of Medicine and Public Health, 2020 County Health Rankings, Social and Economic Factors, accessed May 31, 2020, https://www.countyhealthrankings.org/explore-health-rankings/measures-data-sources/county-health-rankings-model/health-factors/social-and-economic-factors

7   Brad Agnew, "Twentieth-Century Oklahoma," *The Encyclopedia of Oklahoma History and Culture*, https://www.okhistory.org/publications/enc/entry.php?entry=TW001

INFANT MORTALITY RATE

1   Pinterest accessed April 15, 2020, https://www.pinterest.com/pin/159244536799345883/ and www.sayinggoodbye.org

2   J Xu, SL Murphy, KD Kochanek, and E Arias, "Mortality in the United States, 2018," Center for Disease Control and Prevention (CDC), National Center for Health Statistics, NCHS Data Brief, No. 355, January 2020, https://www.cdc.gov/nchs/data/databriefs/db355-h.pdf

3   National Center for Chronic Disease Prevention and Health Promotion, Division of Reproductive Health, "Infant Mortality," accessed December 18, 2020, https://www.cdc.gov/reproductivehealth/maternalinfanthealth/infantmortality.htm

4   DM Ely and AK Driscoll, "Infant Mortality in the United States, 2018: Data from the Period Linked Birth/Infant Death File" National Vital Statistics Reports, Vol 69 No 7, Hyattsville, MD: National Center for Health Statistics, July 16, 2020, https://www.cdc.gov/nchs/data/nvsr/nvsr69/NVSR-69-7-508.pd

5   Oklahoma State Department of Health, "Preparing for a Lifetime, It's Everyone's Responsibility 2019 Snapshot," accessed April 12, 2020, https://oklahoma.gov/content/dam/ok/en/health/health2/documents/p4lt-datasheet-2019.pdf

6   United Health Foundation, "About Infant Mortality" *America's Health Rankings Annual Report 2020*, December 2020, <https://www.americashealthrankings.org/explore/health-of-women-and-children /measure/IMR__MCH/state/>

7   Oklahoma State Department of Health, *State of the State's Health Report*, updated February 26, 2019, https://stateofstateshealth.ok.gov/Data/HealthIndicator

8   March of Dimes, accessed April 9, 2020 at https://www.marchforbabies. org/Registration/mfb2020Signup?utm__source=google&utm__ medium=cpc&utm__campaign=mfb2020&utm__content=brand&utm__ term=march+of+dimes&DonationTrackingParam1=mfb2020__ google&gclid=EAIaIQobChMIj7WsmpTc6AIVAT0MCh1v__wh__ EAAYASAAEgK0RfD__BwE&gclsrc=aw.ds

9   Oklahoma State Department of Health, Maternal and Child Health Service, "Preconception Care and Its Impact on Oklahoma," Oklahoma Pregnancy Risk Assessment Monitoring System (PRAMSGRAM), Vol 14 No 1, Summer 2010, https://www.ok.gov/health2/documents/PramsGram__Preconception%20 Care__%20Summer%202010.pdf

10 Oklahoma State Department of Health, Maternal and Child Health Service, "Maternal Smoking" Oklahoma Pregnancy Risk Assessment Monitoring System (PRAMSGRAM), Vol 9 No 4, 2006, https://oklahoma.gov/content/dam/ok/en/ health/health2/documents/prams-maternal-smoking-06.pdf

11 Oklahoma State Department of Health, Maternal and Child Health Service, "Infant Sleep Position" Oklahoma Pregnancy Risk Assessment Monitoring System (PRAMSGRAM), Vol 11 No 2, Spring 2007, https://www.ok.gov/health2/ documents/PRAMS__Infant%20Sleep%20Position__07.pdf.pdf

12 Oklahoma State Department of Health, accessed April 10, 2020, "Preparing for a Lifetime, It's Everyone's Responsibility," https://www.ok.gov/health/Family__ Health/Improving__Infant__Outcomes/index.html

13 United Health Foundation "About Infant Mortality", 1

14 Oklahoma State Department of Health, Maternal and Child Health Service, "Preconception Care and Its Impact on Oklahoma," 5

15 Oklahoma State Department of Health, Maternal and Child Health Service, "Preconception Care Among Oklahoma Women" *Oklahoma Pregnancy Risk Assessment Monitoring System (PRAMSGRAM)*, Vol 12 No 1, Winter 2008, https:// www.ok.gov/health2/documents/PRAMS__Preconception%20Care__08.pdf

16 Oklahoma State Department of Health, Maternal and Child Health Service, "Disparities in Chronic Health Conditions between Urban and Rural Oklahoma Mothers during the Preconception Period," Oklahoma Pregnancy Risk Assessment Monitoring System (PRAMSGRAM), Vol 21 No 1, May 2019, https://www.ok.gov/ health2/documents/Disparities%20in%20Chronic%20Health%20Conditions%20 (PRAMSgram%20May%202019).pdf

17 J Taylor, C Novoa, K Hamm and S Phadke, *Eliminating Racial Disparities in Maternal and Infant Mortality: A Comprehensive Policy Blueprint*, Washington D.C.: Center for American Progress, May 2, 2019, https://www.americanprogress. org/issues/women/reports/2019/05/02/469186/eliminating-racial-disparities-maternal-infant-mortality/

18 Oklahoma State Department of Health, Maternal and Child Health Service, "Disparities in Chronic Health Conditions between Urban and Rural Oklahoma Mothers during the Preconception Period," 5

19 Taylor, 2-5, 7, 12-14, 26-27, 31, 43-48, and 63-64

20 YA Mohamoud, RS Kirby and DB Ehrenthal, "Poverty, Urban-rural

Classification and Term Infant Mortality: a Population-based Multilevel Analysis," *BMC Pregnancy and Childbirth*, Vol 19 No 40, 2019, https://doi.org/10.1186/s12884-019-2190-1

21 Oklahoma State Department of Health, Maternal and Child Health Service, "Disparities in Chronic Health Conditions between Urban and Rural Oklahoma Mothers during the Preconception Period," 4-5

22 Taylor, 2-5, 7, 12-14, 26-27, 31, 43-48, and 63-64

23 National Center for Chronic Disease Prevention and Health Promotion, Division of Reproductive Health, "Prevention Strategies," accessed April 10, 2020, https://www.cdc.gov/violenceprevention/aces/prevention.html

24 Centers for Disease Control and Prevention, *Preventing Adverse Childhood Experiences: Leveraging the Best Available Evidence*, National Center for Injury Prevention and Control, Centers for Disease Control and Prevention (CDC), Atlanta, GA: 2019, https://www.cdc.gov/violenceprevention/pdf/preventingACES.pdf

25 National Center for Chronic Disease Prevention and Health Promotion, National Center for Injury Prevention and Control, Division of Violence Prevention, *Essentials for Childhood: Creating Safe, Stable, Nurturing Relationships and Environments for All Children*, accessed April 10, 2020, https://www.cdc.gov/violenceprevention/pdf/essentials-for-childhood-framework508.pdf

26 Taylor, 3, 6, 12, 21-23, 26, 28, 30, 39-40, 43-45 and 48-53

27 E Willis, P Mcmanus, N Magallanes and S Johnson, "Conquering Racial Disparities in Perinatal Outcomes" *Clinics in Perinatology*, Vol 41 No. 4, Dec, 2014, https://www.researchgate.net/publication/266619778__Conquering__Racial__Disparities__in__Perinatal__Outcomes

28 C Rogers, FJ Floyd, M Mailick-Seltzer, J Greenberg, and J Hong, "Long-Term Effects of the Death of a Child on Parents' Adjustment in Midlife" *Journal of Family Psychology*, Vol 22 No 2, April 2008, https://www.ncbi.nlm.nih.gov/pmc/articles/PMC2841012/

29 TJ Mathews, MF MacDorman and ME Thoma, "Infant Mortality Statistics from the 2013 Period Linked Birth/Infant Death Data Set, National Vital Statistics Reports, Vol 64 No 9, August 2015, https://www.cdc.gov/nchs/data/nvsr/nvsr64/nvsr64__09.pdf

30 United Health Foundation, "About Infant Mortality," 1

31 Brooke Frye, "Infant Mortality Statistics and Prevention," SUWANNEE RIVER Area Health Education Center, September 2018, https://srahec.org/infant-mortality/?gclid=EAIaIQobChMIk72pgpDc6AIVDlYMCh2__dA3XEAMYAiAAEgLS4PD__Bw)E

32 M Bryant and J Raymond, "Autopsies Reveal a March of Infant Deaths Tied to Unsafe Sleeping" *Oklahoma Watch*, August 2017, https://oklahomawatch.org/2017/08/25/autopsies-reveal-a-march-of-infant-deaths-tied-to-unsafe-sleeping/

33 TJ Mathews, MF MacDorman and ME Thoma, "Infant Mortality Statistics from the 2010 Period Linked Birth/Infant Death Data Set," National Vital Statistics Reports, Vol 62 No 8, December 2013, https://www.cdc.gov/nchs/data/nvsr/nvsr62/nvsr62__08.pdf

34 TJ Mathews, MF MacDorman and ME Thoma, "Infant Mortality Statistics from the 2013 Period Linked Birth/Infant Death Data Set, National Vital Statistics Reports, Vol 64 No 9, August 2015, https://www.cdc.gov/nchs/data/nvsr/nvsr64/nvsr64_09.pdf

35 United Health Foundation, "About Infant Mortality," 1

36 TJ Mathews, MF MacDorman and ME Thoma, "Infant Mortality Statistics from the 2010 Period Linked Birth/Infant Death Data Set," National Vital Statistics Reports, Vol 62 No 8, December 2013, https://www.cdc.gov/nchs/data/nvsr/nvsr62/nvsr62_08.pdf

37 Oklahoma State Department of Health, Maternal and Child Health Service, "Association between Mother's Age at First Birth and Education" *Oklahoma Pregnancy Risk Assessment Monitoring System* (*PRAMSGRAM*), Vol 1, Spring 1995, https://www.ok.gov/health2/documents/PRAMS_Age%20at%20First%20Birth_95.pdf.pdf

38 Oklahoma State Department of Health, "Preparing for a Lifetime, It's Everyone's Responsibility 2019 Snapshot," 1

39 J M Lorenz, C V Ananth, RA Polin and ME D'Alton, " Infant mortality in the United States," *Journal of Perinatology*, Vol 36 No 4, October 2016, https://pubmed.ncbi.nlm.nih.gov/27101388/ DOI https://doi.org/10.1038/jp.2016.63

40 Willis, 847, 852, 855-857, 866 and 869

41 N Racine, A Plamondon, S Madigan, S McDonald and S Tough, "Maternal Adverse Childhood Experiences and Infant Development" *Pediatrics*, Vol 141, No 4, April 2018, https://pediatrics.aappublications.org/content/pediatrics/141/4/e20172495.full.pdf DOI: 10.1542/peds.2017-2495

42 YA Mohamoud, RS Kirby and DB Ehrenthal, "Poverty, urban-rural classification and term infant mortality: a population-based multilevel analysis," 3-4, 6 and 8-10

43 Oklahoma State Department of Health, "Preparing for a Lifetime, It's Everyone's Responsibility 2019 Snapshot," 1

44 Brainy quote, accessed December 21, 2020, https://www.brainyquote.com/quotes/p_j_orourke_617531

CANCER DEATHS

1   Pinterest accessed December 4, 2020, https://www.pinterest.com/pin/425730971007187011/

2   Centers for Disease Control and Prevention (CDC). *An Update on Cancer Deaths in the United States*. Atlanta, GA: US Department of Health and Human Services, Centers for Disease Control and Prevention, Division of Cancer Prevention and Control; Last Reviewed May 29,2020, https://www.cdc.gov/cancer/dcpc/research/update-on-cancer-deaths/

3   Center for Disease Control and Prevention, National Center for Health Statistics, "Cancer Mortality by State" Last reviewed April 29, 2020, https://www.cdc.gov/nchs/pressroom/sosmap/cancer_mortality/cancer.htm

4   U.S. Cancer Statistics Working Group. U.S. Cancer Statistics Data Visualizations Tool, based on 2019 submission data (1999-2017): "Leading Cancer Cases and Deaths, All Races/Ethnicities, Male and Female, 2017" U.S. Department of Health and Human Services, Centers for Disease Control and Prevention (CDC) and National Cancer Institute, released June 2020, https://gis.cdc.gov/Cancer/USCS/DataViz.html

5   American Cancer Society, *Cancer Facts & Figures 2020*, Atlanta: American Cancer Society, 2020, https://www.cancer.org/content/dam/cancer-org/research/cancer-facts-and-statistics/annual-cancer-facts-and-figures/2020/cancer-facts-and-figures-2020.pdf

6   National Cancer Institute, "Risk Factors for Cancer" accessed December 4, 2020, https://www.cancer.gov/about-cancer/causes-prevention/risk

7   American Cancer Society, 1-2, 11, 13-17, 19-28, 30-31, 37, 39-40, 44, 50-52, 56, 59, and 62-64

8   United Health Foundation, "About Cancer," *America's Health Rankings 2020 Annual Report*, December 2020, https://www.americashealthrankings.org/explore/annual/measure/Other__Cancer/state/ALL

9   Centers for Disease Control and Prevention, "How to Prevent Cancer or Find It Early" accessed July 1, 2020, https://www.cdc.gov/cancer/dcpc/prevention/

10 American Cancer Society, 9, 36, 40, 50-54, 59-60, 64 and 66-67

11 Oklahoma Comprehensive Care Network, "It's Our Story to Write: Oklahoma Cancer Prevention and Control Plan 2017-2022" May 2018, https://www.ok.gov/health2/documents/State%20Cancer%20Plan%202017-2022%20updated%20May%2010%202018.pdf

12 KI Alcaraz, TL Wiedt, EC Daniels, KR Yabroff, CE Guerra, and RC Wender, "Understanding and addressing social determinants to advance cancer health equity in the United States: A blueprint for practice, research, and policy" CA: *A Cancer Journal for Clinicians*, Vol 70 No 1, January/February 2020, https://acsjournals.onlinelibrary.wiley.com/doi/full/10.3322/caac.21586

13 United Health Foundation, 1

14 National Cancer Institute, "State Cancer Profiles," accessed July 2, 2020, https://statecancerprofiles.cancer.gov/quick-profiles/index.php?tabSelected=2&statename=oklahoma#t=4

15 S Simon, "Facts & Figures 2019: US Cancer Death Rate has Dropped 27% in 25 Years," American Cancer Society, January 2019, https://www.cancer.org/latest-news/facts-and-figures-2019.html

16 American Cancer Society, 52, 66

17 Oklahoma Comprehensive Care Network, 34

SUICIDE DEATH RATE

1   Rheana Murray, "What is it like to survive a suicide attempt?" *TODAY*, Updated September 23, 2019, https://www.today.com/specials/suicide-attempt-survivors

2   United Health Foundation, "Suicide," *America's Health Rankings Annual Report*, December 2020, https://assets.americashealthrankings.org/app/uploads/ahr-annual-report-2020.pdf https://www.americashealthrankings.org/explore/annual/measure/Suicide/state/OK

3   American Foundation for Suicide Prevention, 1

4   DM Stone, KM Holland, B Bartholow, AE Crosby, S Davis and N Wilkins, *Preventing Suicide A Technical Package of Policy, Programs and Practices*, Atlanta, GA: National Center for Injury Prevention and Control, Centers for Disease Control and Prevention (CDC), 2017, https://www.cdc.gov/violenceprevention/pdf/suicidetechnicalpackage.pdf

5   United Health Foundation, "About Suicide," *America's Health Rankings Annual Report 2020*, December 2020, https://www.americashealthrankings.org/explore/annual/measure/Suicide/state/ALL https://www.americashealthrankings.org/explore/annual/measure/Suicide/state/OK

6   Stone, 12, 19-21, 27, 29, 31-33, 35-36, 38-39 and 58-59

7   Stone, 12 and 15-17

8   DL Steelsmith, CA Fontanella, JV Campo, JA Bridge, KL Warren, and ED Root, "Contextual Factors Associated with County-Level Suicide Rates in the United States, 1999 to 2016" JAMA Network Open. Vol 2 No 9, September 2019, https://jamanetwork.com/journals/jamanetworkopen/fullarticle/2749451, e1910936, doi:10.1001/jamanetworkopen.2019.10936

9   C Bambra, JM Cairns, A Chandler, E Heins, O Kirtley, D McDaid, R O'Connor, and K Smith, "Dying from inequality: Socioeconomic Disadvantage and Suicidal Behaviour", Samaritans, 2017, https://media.samaritans.org/documents/Samaritans__Dying__from__inequality__report__-__summary.pdf

10 United Health Foundation, "Suicide in Oklahoma," *America's Health Rankings Annual Report 2020*, December 2020, https://www.americashealthrankings.org/explore/annual/measure/Suicide/state/OK United Health Foundation, "Suicide in Oklahoma," America's Health Rankings Annual Report 2020, December 2020, https://www.americashealthrankings.org/explore/annual/measure/Suicide/state/OK

11 Stone, 8

12 Oklahoma State Department of Health, "Oklahoma Youth and Young Adult Suicide Report 2020," accessed June 21, 2020, https://www.ok.gov/health2/documents/Youth__And__Young__Adult__Suicide__Report__Oklahoma__2020.pdf

13 National LGBTQ Education Center, *Suicide Risk and Prevention for LGBTQ People*, September 2018, https://www.lgbtqiahealtheducation.org/wp-content/uploads/2018/10/Suicide-Risk-and-Prevention-for-LGBTQ-Patients-Brief.pdf

14 United Health Foundation, "About Suicide," 1

15 Stone, 8 and 26

16 American Foundation for Suicide Prevention, "Risk Factors and Warning Signs" accessed June 21, 2020, https://afsp.org/risk-factors-and-warning-signs

17 Stone, 8, 9 and 19

18 America's Health Rankings, "About Suicide" 1

19 Stone, 8-9, 19 and 47

20 Stone, 15 and 19

21 JA Hoffman, CA Farrell, MC Monuteaux, "Pediatric Suicide Rates and Community-Level Poverty in the United States, 2007-2016," American Academy of Pediatrics, October 2019, https://services.aap.org/en/news-room/news-releases/aap/2019/study-finds-youth-suicide-rates-rise-with-community-poverty-levels/

22 America's Health Rankings, "About Suicide," 1

23 WC Kerr, MS Kaplan, N Huguet, R Caetano, N Ciesbrecht, and BH McFarland, "Economic Recession, Alcohol, and Suicide Rates: Comparative Effects of Poverty, Foreclosure, and Job Loss," American Journal of Preventive Medicine, April 2017, https://www.ajpmonline.org/article/S0749-3797(16)30461-5/fulltext

24 Bambra, 5-12, 15-16, 20-22, and 24-25

25 Suicide Prevention Lifeline, "We Can All Prevent Suicide," accessed June 22, 2020, https://suicidepreventionlifeline.org/how-we-can-all-prevent-suicide/

ADDICTION AND DRUG DEATHS

1 S San Filippo, "Love What Matters," accessed December 7, 2020, https://www.lovewhatmatters.com/a-guardian-angel-called-9-1-1-as-i-convulsed-in-a-coffee-shop-addiction-prison-recovery-alcoholism-sober-hope-lung-cancer-kindness/

2 National Institute on Drug Abuse (NIDA), "Oklahoma: Opioid-Involved Death and Related Harms," April 2020, https://www.drugabuse.gov/opioid-summaries-by-state/oklahoma-opioid-involved-deaths-related-harms

3 United Health Foundation, "Drug Deaths" *America's Health Rankings Annual Report 2020*, December 2020, https://assets.americashealthrankings.org/app/uploads/annual20-rev-complete.pdf

4 Oklahoma State Department of Health, Injury Prevention Service, "Drug Overdose," accessed December 28, 2020, https://oklahoma.gov/health/prevention-and-preparedness/injury-prevention-service/drug-overdose.html

5 Centers for Disease Control, "2018 Drug Overdose Death Rates," March 10, 2020, https://www.cdc.gov/drugoverdose/data/statedeaths/drug-overdose-death-2018.html

6 Jaclyn Cosgrove, "Cost of addiction in Oklahoma," *The Oklahoman*, March 10, 2012, https://oklahoman.com/article/3656381/cost-of-addiction-in-oklahoma-an-estimated-72-billion-per-year

7 Office of the Attorney General, "Oklahoma Commission on Opioid Abuse Final Report," December 31, 2019, https://www.oag.ok.gov/sites/g/files/gmc766/f/documents/2020/opioid__report__2019__-__annual__report.pdf

8 United Health Foundation, "Drug Deaths," 37 and 39

9 United Health Foundation, "Health Insurance" *America's Health Ranking Annual Report 2020*, December 2020, https://assets.americashealthrankings.org/app/uploads/annual20-rev-complete.pdf

10 Beach House Treatment, "Addiction: Why Doctors and Pilots Recover at Much Higher Rates," February 28, 2020, https://beachhousetreatment.com/addiction-why-doctors-and-pilots-recover-at-much-higher-rates/

11 United Health Foundation, "About Drug Deaths," *America's Health Rankings Annual Report 2020*, December 2020, https://www.americashealthrankings.org/explore/annual/measure/drug__deaths__1yr/state/OK

12 Office of Attorney General, 9

13 JJ Carroll, TC Green, and RK Noonan, "Evidence-Based Strategies for Preventing Opioid Overdose: What's Working in the United States, 2018," Centers for Disease Control and Prevention (CDC), National Center for Injury Prevention and Control, 2018, http://www. cdc.gov/drugoverdose/pdf/pubs/2018-evidence-based-strategies.pdf

14 Centers for Disease Control and Prevention, National Center for Injury Prevention and Control, Division of Violence Prevention, "Preventing Adverse Childhood Experiences (ACEs): Leveraging the Best Available Evidence", Atlanta, GA: 2019, https://www.cdc.gov/violenceprevention/pdf/preventingACES.pdf

15 Office of the Attorney General, 9

16 National Institute on Drug Abuse (NIDA), 1

17 National Institute on Drug Abuse (NIDA), 1

18 Consumer Reports, Inc., "Many people fail to get rid of unneeded and expired drugs" *Washington Post*, July 23, 2018, https://www.washingtonpost.com/national/health-science/many-people-fail-to-get-rid-of-unneeded-and-expired-drugs/2018/07/20/0c87e024-65d6-11e8-a768-ed043e33f1dc__story.html

19 Brainy Quote, accessed December 7, 2020, https://www.brainyquote.com/quotes/oprah__winfrey__103803

20 Anonymous, "My recovery must come first so that everything I love in life doesn't have to come last," Willow Springs Recovery, accessed December 7, 2020, https://www.willowspringsrecovery.com/recovery/40-quotes-to-inspire-addiction-recovery/

TOBACCO

1 The Quotes Master, accessed December 22, 2020, http://thequotesmaster.com/2015/12/660/

2 Oklahoma State Department of Health, Center for Chronic Disease Prevention & Health Promotion, "Oklahoma State Plan: 150,000 Fewer Tobacco Users by 2022," Revised December 2019, https://www.ok.gov/health2/documents/2019%20-%20OK%20State%20Plan%20for%20Tobacco%20Use%20Prevention%20%20Cessation.pdf

3 United Health Foundation, "Smoking," *America's Health Rankings Annual Report 2020*, December 2020, https://assets.americashealthrankings.org/app/uploads/annual20-rev-complete.pdf

4 Oklahoma State Department of Health, 9

5 United Health Foundation, "About Smoking," *America's Health Rankings Annual Report 2020*, December 2020, https://www.americashealthrankings.org/explore/annual/measure/Smoking/state/ALL

6 Oklahoma State Department of Health, 6 and 12

7 American Cancer Society, *Cancer Facts & Figures 2020*, Atlanta: American Cancer Society, 2020, https://www.cancer.org/content/dam/cancer-org/research/cancer-facts-and-statistics/annual-cancer-facts-and-figures/2020/cancer-facts-and-figures-2020.pdf

8 Oklahoma State Department of Health, 16

9 Oklahoma State Department of Health, 20

10 Tobacco Settlement Endowment Fund (TSET), Tobacco Stops with Me "Clearing the Air," accessed June 25, 2020, https://stopswithme.com/not-ok/clean-indoor-air/

11 Tobacco Settlement Endowment Fund (TSET), Tobacco Stops with Me, "Banning Menthol and Flavored Tobacco," accessed June 25, 2020, https://stopswithme.com/not-ok/flavored-tobacco-ban/

12 Oklahoma State Department of Health, 20

13 "Robert Wood Johnson Foundation, "Mass media campaigns against tobacco use," *County Health Rankings & Roadmaps*, April 18, 2019, https://www.countyhealthrankings.org/take-action-to-improve-health/what-works-for-health/strategies/mass-media-campaigns-against-tobacco-use

14 United Health Foundation, "About Smoking," 1

15 Oklahoma State Department of Health, 9

16 Oklahoma State Department of Health, 5-6

17 Center for Disease Control and Prevention (CDC), "Secondhand Smoke (SHS) Facts," accessed June 25, 2020, https://www.cdc.gov/tobacco/data__statistics/ fact__sheets/secondhand__smoke/general__facts/index.htm

18 Oklahoma State Department of Health, 5-6 and 9

19 Center for Disease Control and Prevention (CDC), "Secondhand Smoke (SHS) Facts," 1

20 Center for Disease Control and Prevention (CDC), "Secondhand Smoke (SHS) Facts," 1

21 Centers for Disease Control and Prevention (CDC), "Youth and Tobacco Use," accessed June 25, 2020, https://www.cdc.gov/tobacco/data__statistics/fact__ sheets/youth__data/tobacco__use/index.htm

22 Centers for Disease Control and Prevention (CDC) "Smokeless Tobacco: Health Effects," accessed June 25, 2020, https://www.cdc.gov/tobacco/data__ statistics/fact__sheets/smokeless/health__effects/index.htm

23 Oklahoma State Department of Health, 14

24 Center for Disease Control and Prevention (CDC), "Electronic Cigarettes" accessed June 25, 2020, https://www.cdc.gov/tobacco/basic__information/e-cigarettes/index.htm

25 CBQ Method, accessed June 25, 2020, https:/smokingcessationformula. com/10-quit-smoking-quotes-that-helped-me-quit/

26 Pinterest, accessed December 22, 2020, https://in.pinterest.com/ pin/80150068353026637/

OBESITY

1 Brainy Quote, accessed June 25, 2020, https://www.brainyquote.com/quotes/ tom__vilsack__459330

2 Goodreads, accessed December 9, 2020, https://www.goodreads.com/ quotes/467501-associated-with-this-weight-gain-are-increased-risks-in-adulthood

3 Tobacco Settlement Endowment Program (TSET), "TSET Healthy Living Program," accessed June 25, 2020, https://tset.ok.gov/sites/g/files/gmc166/f/ TSET%20HLP%20Fact%20Sheet%20Update__June-2019.pdf

4 United Health Foundation, "Obesity in Oklahoma," *America's Health Rankings Annual Report 2020*, December 2020, https://www.americashealthrankings.org/ explore/annual/measure/Obesity/state/

5 Robert Wood Johnson Foundation, "Oklahoma," *State of Childhood Obesity, Helping all Children Grow Up Healthy*, accessed December 10, 2020, ‹https:// stateofchildhoodobesity.org/states/ok/› https://stateofchildhoodobesity.org/states/ ok/

6 Trust for America's Health (TFAH), "Oklahoma at a glance," accessed December 10, 2020, https://www.tfah.org/state-details/oklahoma/

7 Oklahoma State Department of Health, *Healthy Oklahoma 2020 Bringing Oklahoma's Health into Focus: Oklahoma Health Improvement Plan*, accessed June 30, 2020, https://www.ok.gov/health2/documents/OHIP%202020.pdff

8 Tobacco Settlement Endowment Trust (TSET), "Healthy Living Program," 1

9 Tobacco Settlement Endowment Trust (TSET) "Shape Your Future," accessed

June 25, 2020, https://shapeyourfutureok.com/overweight-obesitys-impact-oklahoma/health-actions/

10 Oklahoma State Department of Health, Chronic Disease Service, *Get Fit Eat Smart OK, Oklahoma Physical Activity and Nutrition State Plan*, ‹https://www.ok.gov/health2/documents/OKPAN__State__Plan.pdf› https://www.ok.gov/health2/documents/OKPAN__State__Plan.pdf, accessed January 16, 2020

11 Tobacco Settlement Endowment Trust (TSET) "Shape Your Future," 1

12 Trust for America's Health (TFAH), *The State of Obesity 2019: Better Policies for A Healthier America*, September 2019, ‹https://media.stateofobesity.org/ wp-content/uploads/2019/09/16100613/2019Ob esityReportFINAL.pdf› https://media.stateofobesity.org/wp-content/uploads/2019/09/16100613/2019ObesityReportFINAL.pdf

13 Trust for America's Health (TFAH), *The State of Obesity 2020: Better Policies for A Healthier America*, September 2020, ‹https://media.stateofobesity.org/wp-content/uploads/2019/09/16100613/2019Ob esityReportFINAL.pdf› https://media.stateofobesity.org/wp-content/uploads/2019/09/16100613/2019ObesityReportFINAL.pdf

14 Trust for America's Health, *The State of Obesity 2019: Better Policies for A Healthier America*, 5, 8-9, 11, 16-17, 43-46, 50, 53, 55-56, 62-64 and 67-68,

15 Trust for America's Health (TFAH), *The State of Obesity 2020: Better Policies for A Healthier America*, 5-6, 9, 11-14, 20, 22-24, 28-29, 38-39, 44-51, 53-58, 63-65, 68 -73, 78

16 Tobacco Settlement Endowment Trust (TSET) "Shape Your Future," 1

17 SN Bleich, HG Lawman, MT LeVasseur, J Yan, N Mitra, CM Lowery, A Peterhans, S Hua LA Gibson and CA Roberto, "The Association of a Sweetened Beverage Tax with Changes in Beverage Prices and Purchases at Independent Stores" Health Affairs, Vol 39, No 7 July 2020, https://www.healthaffairs.org/doi/10.1377/hlthaff.2019.01058

18 Oklahoma State Department of Health, Center for Chronic Disease Prevention and Health Promotion, "Burden of Obesity in Oklahoma," August 2020, https://www.ok.gov/health2/documents/Burden%20of%20Obesity%20in%20Oklahoma.pdf

19 Harvard University, TH Chan School of Public Health, "Obesity Trends" accessed December 10, 2020, https://www.hsph.harvard.edu/obesity-prevention-source/obesity-trends/

20 United Health Foundation, "Obesity," *America's Health Rankings Annual Report 2020*, December 2020, ‹https://assets.americashealthrankings.org/app/uploads/ahr-annual-report-202 0.pdf› https://assets.americashealthrankings.org/app/uploads/ahr-annual-report-2020 .pdf

21 Oklahoma State Department of Health, "Oklahoma Youth Risk Behavior Survey (YRBS)- 10-Year Trends in Prevalence for Selected Health Indicators: 2009-2019," accessed June 25, 2020, https://www.ok.gov/health2/documents/YRBS__10__Year__Trend__Monitoring__Sheet%202009-2019.pdf

22 Trust for America's Health (TFAH), *The State of Obesity: BETTER POLICIES FOR A HEALTHIER AMERICA 2020*, 37

23 Oklahoma State Department of Health, "Oklahoma Youth Risk Behavior Survey (YRBS)- 10-Year Trends in Prevalence for Selected Health Indicators: 2009-2019," 1).

24 OPRAH.COM, accessed June 25, 2020, http://www.oprah.com/quote/lidia-yuknavitch-quote-beauty

INCARCERATION

1   Goodreads, accessed December 11, 2020, https://www.goodreads.com/author/show/57926.Mumia__Abu__

2   P Wagner and W Bertram, "What percent of the U.S. is incarcerated?" (And other ways to measure mass incarceration)" Prison Policy Initiative, January 16, 2020, https://www.prisoner.org/blog/2020/01/16/percent-incarcerated/

3   EA Carson, "Prisoners in 2019" U.S. Department of Justice, Bureau of Justice Statistics, October 2020, https://www.bjs.gov/index.cfm?ty=pbdetail&iid=7106

4   Oklahoma Justice Reform Task Force, "Oklahoma Justice Reform Task Force Final Report," February 2017, https://www.ok.gov/dcs/searchdocs/app/manage__documents.php?att__id=22034

5   S Becker and L Alexander, "Understanding the Impacts of Incarceration on Health: A Framework," ReThink Health, March 2016, https://www.rethinkhealth.org/wp-content/uploads/2016/04/ReThink-Health-March-17-Report-1.pdf

6   Healthy People 2020, "Incarceration," accessed June 9, 2020, https://www.healthypeople.gov/2020/topics-objectives/topic/social-determinants-health/interventions-resources/incarceration

7   Oklahoma Justice Reform Task Force, 23

8   Becker, 5 and 7

9   S Sharp, S Marcus-Mendoza, R Bentley, D Simpson and S Love, "Gender Differences in the Impact of Incarceration on the Children and Families of Drug Offenders", Journal of the Oklahoma Criminal Justice Research Consortium, January 1999, Vol. 4, https://www.researchgate.net/publication/253935089__Gender__Differences__in__the__Impact__of__Incarceration__on__the__Children__and__Families__of__Drug__Offenders

10 Becker, 3-6, 8 and 12

11   D Shade, "The Governor's justice task force gives lawmakers a chance to address the scale of Oklahoma's prison crisis," Oklahoma Policy Institute, Updated January 12, 2020, https://okpolicy.org/the-governors-justice-task-force-gives-lawmakers-a-chance-to-address-the-scale-of-oklahomas-prison-crisis/

12 Oklahoma Department of Mental Health and Substance Abuse, "Adult Drug Court," accessed June 9, 2020, https://www.ok.gov/odmhsas/Substance__Abuse/Oklahoma__Drug__and__Mental__Health__Courts/Adult__Drug__Court/index.html

13 Shade, 1

14 A Harvey, "It's time to restructure Oklahoma courts' wildly inefficient and unjust fines and fees system," Oklahoma Policy Institute, March 16, 2020, https://okpolicy.org/its-time-to-restructure-oklahoma-courts-wildly-inefficient-and-unjust-fines-and-fees-system/

15 Oklahoma State Department of Mental Health and Substance Abuse, 1

16 Oklahomans for Criminal Justice Reform, "Oklahoma's Imprisonment Crisis, 2019 Legislative Agenda," accessed April 19, 2020, https://okjusticereform.org/wp-content/uploads/2019/02/ok__OCJR__Agenda-v4.pdf

17 R Genzler, "SB 252 bail reform could save counties & communities millions," Oklahoma Policy Institute, Open Justice Oklahoma, accessed April 19, 2020, https://openjustice.okpolicy.org/wp-content/uploads/sites/4/2019/02/Bail-Fact-Sheet-2019-Summary-Final.pdf?x67581

18 S Lewis, "The cost of maintaining the world's highest incarceration (Capitol Update)" Oklahoma Policy Institute, Updated May 2, 2019, https://okpolicy.org/the-cost-of-maintaining-the-worlds-highest-incarceration-capitol-update/

19 A Nellis, "The Color of Justice: Racial and Ethnic Disparity in State Prisons," The Sentencing Project, June 2016, https://www.sentencingproject.org/publications/color-of-justice-racial-and-ethnic-disparity-in-state-prisons/

20 Becker, 2 and 5-7

21 Sharp, 1-3, 5 and 8-13

22 Pass It On, accessed December 11, 2020, https://www.passiton.com/inspirational-quotes/7395

TEEN BIRTH RATE

1 Accessed June 19, 2020, https://www.smith.edu/ourhealthourfutures/teenpreg6.html

2 The American College of Obstetricians and Gynecologists (ACOG), Committee on Adolescent Health Care, "Adolescent Pregnancy, Contraception, and Sexual Activity" No. 699, May 2017, Reaffirmed 2019, https://www.acog.org/clinical/clinical-guidance/committee-opinion/articles/2017/05/adolescent-pregnancy-contraception-and-sexual-activity

3 Oklahoma State Department of Health, Maternal and Child Health Assessment, "Oklahoma Teen Birth Rate: 1994-2018," December 2019, https://Oklahoma.gov/content/dam/ok/en/health/health2/documents/oklahoma-teen-birth-report-1994-2018.pdf

4 JA Martin, BE Hamilton, MJK Osterman and AK Driscoll, "Births: Final Data for 2018," National Vital Statistics Reports; Hyattsville, MD: National Center for Health Statistics. Vol 68 No 13, November 27, 2019, https://www.cdc.gov/nchs/data/nvsr68/nvsr68__13-508.pdf

5 Oklahoma State Department of Health, "Oklahoma's State of the State's Health," accessed June 19, 2020, https://stateofstateshealth.ok.gov/Data/HealthIndicator

6 Center for Disease Control and Prevention (CDC), "CDC Vital Signs Preventing Teen Pregnancy: A key role for health care providers," April 2015, https://www.cdc.gov/vitalsigns/pdf/2015-04-vitalsigns.pdf

7 Oklahoma State Department of Health, Maternal & Child Health Service/Child & Adolescent Health Division, "Teen Pregnancy Prevention: What can Youth Serving Organizations Do?" Accessed December 12, 2020, https://www.ok.gov/health2/documents/What%20You%20Can%20Do%20-%20Youth%20Serving%20Organizations.pdf

8 Centers for Disease Control and Prevention (CDC) Division of Reproductive Health, "Teen Pregnancy: About Teen Pregnancy," January 10, 2019, https://www.cdc.gov/teenpregnancy/about/index.htm

9 Oklahoma State Department of Health, Maternal & Child Health Service/Child & Adolescent Health Division, "Teen Pregnancy Prevention: What can Schools Do?," accessed December 12, 2020, https://www.ok.gov/health2/documents/What%20You%20Can%20Do%20-%20Schools.pdf

10 Centers for Disease Control and Prevention (CDC), Division of Adolescent and School Health (DASH), "What Works: Sexual Health Education" February 3,

2020, https://www.cdc.gov/healthyyouth/whatworks/what-works-sexual-health-education.htm

11 The American College of Obstetricians and Gynecologists (ACOG), 2, 5

12 Planned Parenthood Federation of America, "Reducing Teenage Pregnancy," July 2013, https://www.plannedparenthood.org/files/6813/9611/7632/Reducing__Teen__Pregnancy.pdf

13 Centers for Disease Control and Prevention (CDC), Division of Reproductive Health, "Teen Pregnancy: Social Determinants and Eliminating Disparities in Teen Pregnancy" October 15, 2019, https://www.cdc.gov/teenpregnancy/about/social-determinants-disparities-teen-pregnancy.htm

14 Centers for Disease Control and Prevention (CDC), Division of Reproductive Health, "Teen Pregnancy: Projects and Initiatives, March 26, 2018, https://www.cdc.gov/teenpregnancy/projects-initiatives/index.html

15 Oklahoma State Department of Health, "Adolescent Sexual Health in Oklahoma 2019," accessed December 17, 2020, https://oklahoma.gov/content/dam/ok/en/health/health2/docs/Adolescent__Sexual__Health__Report__Oklahoma__2019%20(1).pdf

16 Oklahoma State Department of Health, "Adolescent Sexual Health in Oklahoma 2019,"4

17 Oklahoma State Department of Health, "Oklahoma Youth Risk Behavior Survey (YRBS)- 10-Year Trends in Prevalence for Selected Health Indicators: 2009-2019," accessed December 17, 2020, https://oklahoma.gov/content/dam/ok/en/health/health2/documents/yrbs-10-year-trend-monitoring-sheet-2009-2019.pdf

18 Power to Decide, "Progress Pays Off, January 2018, https://powertodecide.org/sites/default/files/cost-fact-sheets/savings-fact-sheet-OK.pdf

19 Mayo Clinic, "Tween and Teen Health" accessed June 18, 2020, https://www.mayoclinic.org/healthy-lifestyle/tween-and-teen-health/in-depth/teen-pregnancy/art-20048124

20 Centers for Disease Control and Prevention (CDC) Division of Reproductive Health, "Teen Pregnancy: Social Determinants and Eliminating Disparities in Teen Pregnancy," 1

21 JM Zweig and E Falkenburger, "Poverty, Vulnerability, and the Safety Net" Urban Institute, Urban Wire (put in blog format) September 6, 2017, https://www.urban.org/urban-wire/preventing-teen-pregnancy-can-help-prevent-poverty

22 QuoteHD.com, accessed June 19, 2020, http://www.quotehd.com/quotes/jordan-brown-quote-reducing-teen-pregnancy-and-birth-is-one-of-the-most

23 Boston's Children Hospital accessed March 19, 2021 at https://thriving.childrenshospital.org/lifetime-movie-based-on-alleged-teen-pregnancy-pact/

POVERTY

1 Grimes, Shaunta, "What Poor Feels Like" Huff Post, March 15, 2017, https://www.huffpost.com/entry/what-poor-feels-like__b__58c96165e4b022994fa3e8b0

2 B Butrica, K Martinchek, MM. Galvez, H Hahn, SM McKernan and S Spaulding, Effective Programs and Policies Promoting Economic Well-Being: Lessons from the Financial Security, Housing, Workforce Development, and Case Management Fields," Urban Institute, February, 2020, urban Institute; Retrieved

February 24 2020 at https://www.urban.org/research/publication/effective-programs-and-policies-promoting-economic-well-being

3   United States Census Bureau, "Poverty Status in the Past 12 Months" 2019: American Community Survey (ACS) 1-Year Estimates Subject Tables, TableID: S1701, accessed December 13, 2020, https://data.census.gov/cedsci/table?q=poverty%20oklahoma%20and%20united%20states&tid=ACSST1Y2019.S1701&hidePreview=false

4   United Health Foundation, "High School Graduation," *America's Health Rankings 2020*, December 2020, <https://assets.americashealthrankings.org/app/uploads/annual20-rev-complete .pdf> https://assets.americashealthrankings.org/app/uploads/annual20-rev-complete.d-children/state-summaries-oklahoma

5   The Annie E. Casey Foundation., *The 2020 KIDS COUNT Data Book: State Trends in Child Well-Being*, © 2020, Baltimore, Maryland: The Annie E. Casey Foundation, June 22, 2020, www.aecf.org/databook

6   R Fine, "Black and Latino children in Oklahoma are still more likely to live in concentrated poverty," Oklahoma Policy Institute, October 4, 2019, https://okpolicy.org/black-and-latino-children-in-oklahoma-are-still-more-likely-to-live-in-concentrated-poverty/

7   The Annie E. Casey Foundation., "Children Living in High-Poverty, Low-Opportunity Neighborhoods" © 2019, Baltimore, Maryland: The Annie E. Casey Foundation, September 24, 2019, https://www.aecf.org/resources/children-living-in-high-poverty-low-opportunity-neighborhoods

8   T Frohlich, MB. Sauter and A Kent, "Progress in fighting poverty in America has slowed despite recent economic recovery" USA Today, October 4, 2018, https://www.usatoday.com/story/money/economy/2018/10/01/fighting-poverty-america-slowing-despite-recent-economic-recovery/1445296002/

9   The Annie E. Casey Foundation, "Kids in Concentrated Poverty Data Snapshot, September 24, 2019, https://www.aecf.org/blog/percentage-of-kids-in-concentrated-poverty-worsens-in-10-states-and-puerto/

10 Virginia Commonwealth University Center on Society and Health, "Education: It Matters More to Health than Ever Before," February 13, 2015, https://societyhealth.vcu.edu/work/the-projects/education-it-matters-more-to-health-than-ever-before.htm

11 Butrica, 1-4, 12, 22, 25-28, 33-34, 37—42, 46-47, 56-57, 61, 64-66 and 74-75

12 Task Force on the Future of Higher Education, "Report on the Future of Higher Education," February 2018, https://www.okhighered.org/future/docs/final-report.pdf

13 C Cullison, "Smart policy decisions could improve economic well-being for all Oklahomans," Oklahoma Policy Institute, February 24, 2020, https://okpolicy.org/smart-policy-decisions-could-improve-economic-well-being-for-all-oklahomans/

14 Butrica, 25, 37 and 42

15 The Annie E. Casey Foundation, *The 2020 KIDS COUNT Data Book*, 1, 20 and 36

16 R Fine, 1

17 C Cullison, "It's Poverty Week at OK Policy – here's what to expect," Oklahoma Policy Institute, September 23, 2019, https://okpolicy.org/its-poverty-week-at-ok-policy-heres-what-to-expect/

18 Butrica, 1-4, 12, 22, 25-28, 31, 33-34, 37-42, 46-47, 56-57, 61, 64-66 and 74-75

19 Frohlich, 1

20 AZ Quotes, accessed June 27, 2020, https://www.azquotes.com/quotes/topics/health-and-education.html

EDUCATION

1 Quotefancy, accessed December 14, 2020, https://quotefancy.com/quote/1601250/Joycelyn-Elders-I-feel-that-we-can-t-educate-children-who-are-not-healthy-and-we-can-t

2 Virginia Commonwealth University Center on Society and Health, Education and Health Initiative, "We all know that a good education is important," Updated December 9, 2020, https://societyhealth.vcu.edu/work/the-projects/educationhealth.html

3 National Center for Education Statistics, Digest of Education Statistics "Table 219.46. Public high school 4-year adjusted cohort graduation rate (ACGR), by selected student characteristics and state: 2010-11 through 2017-18," February, 2020, https://nces.ed.gov/programs/digest/d19/tables/dt19__219.46.asp

4 United Health Foundation, "High School Graduation," America's Health Rankings 2020, December 2020, https://assets.americashealthrankings.org/app/uploads/annual20-rev-complete.pdf

5 MN Atwell, R Balfanz, E Manspile, V Byrnes and J Bridgeland, "Building a Grad Nation: Progress and Challenge in Raising High School Graduation Rates Annual Update 2020," Civic, John Hopkins University, Everyone Graduates Center at the School of Education, accessed December 29, 2020, https://www.americaspromise.org/report/2020-building-grad-nation-report

6 US News and World Report, "Best States," accessed December 15, 2020, https://www.usnews.com/news/best-states/oklahoma

7 US Census Bureau, " Educational Attainment, 2019: American Community Survey (ACS) 1-Year Estimates Subject Tables TableID: S1501, accessed December 14, 2020, https://data.census.gov/cedsci/table?q=educational attainment us and oklahoma&tid=ACSST1Y2019.S1501&hidePreview=false

8 Oklahoma Works, "Launch Oklahoma Strategic Plan," November 2017, https://oklahomaworks.gov/wp-content/uploads/2017/04/Launch-OK-Strategic-Recommendations-2017.pdf

9 AP Carnevale, TI Garcia, N Ridley and MC Quinn, "The Overlooked Value of Certificates and Associate's Degrees: What Students need to Know Before they go to College, Georgetown University Center on Education and the Workforce, January 2020, https://1gyhoq479ufd3yna29x7ubjn-wpengine.netdna-ssl.com/wp-content/uploads/CEW-SubBA.pdf

10 Virginia Commonwealth University Center on Society and Health, Education and Health Initiative, "Why Education Matters to Health: Exploring the Causes," Accessed June 23, 2020, https://societyhealth.vcu.edu/media/society-health/pdf/test-folder/CSH-EHI-Issue-Brief-2.pdf

11 Office of Disease Prevention and Health Promotion, Healthy People 2020, "Social Determinants of Health," accessed December 14, 2020, https://www.healthypeople.gov/2020/topics-objectives/topic/social-determinants-of-health

12 M Atwell, Robert Balfanz, J Bridgeland, and E Ingram, "Building a Grad Nation:

Progress and Challenge in Raising High School Graduation Rates Annual Update 2019, Civic, John Hopkins University, Everyone Graduates Center at the School of Education, accessed June 23, 2020, https://www.americaspromise.org/2019-building-grad-nation-report

13 Atwell, "Building a Grad Nation: Annual Update 2020," 9-10, 12, 16, 32-33 and 35-36

14 <https://www.edweek.org/by/catherine-gewertz> C Gewertz, "The Challenge of Creating Schools That 'Work for Everybody," *Education Week*, March 21, 2017, <https://www.edweek.org/teaching-learning/the-challenge-of-creating-schools-that-work-for-everybody/2017/03> https://www.edweek.org/teaching-learning/the-challenge-of-creating-schools-that-work-for-everybody/2017/03

15 S Sandoval, "How Our District Reimagined Special Education," *Education Week*, September 17, 2019, <https://www.edweek.org/leadership/opinion-how-our-district-reimagined-special-education/2019/09> https://www.edweek.org/leadership/opinion-how-our-district-reimagined-special-education/2019/09

16 J Taylor, C Novoa, K Hamm and S Phadke, *Eliminating Racial Disparities in Maternal and Infant Mortality: A Comprehensive Policy Blueprint*. Washington D.C.: Center for American Progress, May 2, 2019, https://www.americanprogress.org/issues/women/reports/2019/05/02/469186/eliminating-racial-disparities-maternal-infant-mortality/

17 American Public Health Association (APHA), "School-Based Health Centers: Improving Health, Well-being and Educational Success," February 2018, https://www.apha.org/-/media/files/pdf/sbhc/well__being__in__schools.ashx?la=en&hash=F54F7A314E6EB201C8B91F0EF8DDC673E6A35187

18 Task Force on the Future of Higher Education, "Report on the Future of Higher Education," February 2018, https://www.okhighered.org/future/docs/final-report.pdf

19 Virginia Commonwealth University, Center on Society and Health, "Education: It Matters More to Health than Ever Before," 1-5

20 Virginia Commonwealth University, Center on Society and Health, "Why Education Matters to Health: Exploring the Causes," 2

21 Virginia Commonwealth University, Center on Society and Health, "Education: It Matters More to Health than Ever Before," 5-6

22 Office of Disease Prevention and Health Promotion, Healthy People 2020, "Social Determinants of Health," 1

23 B DeBaun and M Roc, "Well and Well-Off: Decreasing Medicaid and Health-Care Costs by Increasing Educational Attainment" Alliance for Excellence in Education (all4ed), July 10, 2013, https://mk0all4edorgjxiy8xf9.kinstacdn.com/wp-content/uploads/2013/08/WellWellOff.pdf

24 DeBaun, "Well and Well-Off," 7

25 Atwell, Building a Grad Nation: Annual Update 2020," 50

26 Virginia Commonwealth University Center on Society and Health, "Education: It Matters More to Health than Ever Before," 1

27 Virginia Commonwealth University Center on Society and Health, "Why Education Matters to Health: Exploring the Causes," 3

28 Office of Disease Prevention and Health Promotion, Healthy People 2020, "Social Determinants of Health," 1

29 Brainy Quote, accessed September 15, 2020, https://www.brainyquote.com/quotes/buzz__aldrin__179474

UNINSURED

1 Brainy Quote, accessed June 29, 2020, https://www.brainyquote.com/quotes/colin__powell__411915

2 J Tolbert, K Orgera, and A. Damico, "Key Facts about the Uninsured Population," Kaiser Family Foundation (KFF), November 6, 2020, https:/www.kff.org/uninsured/issue-brief/key-facts-about-the-uninsured-population/

3 E. Ward, M Halpern, NM Marlow, V Cokkinides, C DeSantis, P Bandi, R Siegel, A Stewart, and A Jemal, "Association of Insurance with Cancer Care Utilization and Outcomes", ‹https://www.researchgate.net/journal/CA-A-Cancer-Journal-for-Clinicians-0007-9235› CA *A Cancer Journal for Clinicians* Volume 58 No. 1, January/February 2008, https://acsjournals.onlinelibrary.wiley.com/doi/full/10.3322/CA.2007.0011

4 R Garfield, K Orgera and A Damico, "The Uninsured and the ACA: A Primer: Key Facts about Health Insurance and the Uninsured amidst Changes to the Affordable Care Act" Kaiser Family Foundation (KFF), January 2019, http://files.kff.org/attachment/The-Uninsured-and-the-ACA-A-Primer-Key-Facts-about-Health-Insurance-and-the-Uninsured-amidst-Changes-to-the-Affordable-Care-Act

5 US Census Bureau, "Selected Characteristics of Health Insurance Coverage in the United States, 2019 American Community Survey (ACS) 1-Year Estimates Subject Tables, TableID: S2701, accessed December 16, 2020, https://data.census.gov/cedsci/table?q=2019 uninsured oklahomans&tid=ACSST1Y2019.S2701&hidePreview=false

6 United Health Foundation, "Uninsured," *America's Health Rankings Annual Report 2020*, December 2020, https://assets.americashealthrankings.org/app/uploads/annual20-rev-complete..pdf

7 LJ Blumberg, M Karpman, M Buettgens, and Solleveld, "Who Are the Remaining Uninsured, and What Do Their Characteristics Tell Us About How to Reach Them?," Urban Institute, March 2016, http://www.urban.org/sites/default/files/publication/79051/2000691-Who-Are-The-Remaining-Uninsured-And-What-Do-Their-Characteristics-Tell-Us-About__How-To__Reach__Them.pdf?

8 Tolbert, 1

9 R Tikkanen and Mk Abrams, "U.S. Health Care from a Global Perspective, 2019: Higher Spending, Worse Outcomes, The Commonwealth Fund, January 2020, https://www.commonwealthfund.org/sites/default/files/2020-01/Tikkanen__US__hlt__care__global__perspective__2019__OECD__db__v2.pdf

10 Tikkanen, 2,5,15 and 16

11 United Health Foundation, "Clinical Care," 20

12 Tolbert, 1

13 Ward, 9-10, 19, 21, 23-26, and 28-30

14 United Health Foundation, "Clinical Care," 19-20

15 P Shinn and M Martin, "Medicaid expansion: Ten years of unparalleled return on investment, improved outcomes," Oklahoma Policy Institute, June 24, 2020, https://okpolicy.org/medicaid-expansion-ten-years-of-unparalleled-return-on-investment-improved-outcomes/

16 Kaiser Family Foundation (KFF), "Who Could Medicaid Reach with Expansion in Oklahoma" June 30, 2020, http://files.kff.org/attachment/fact-sheet-medicaid-expansion-OK

17 M Guth, R Garfield, and R Rudowitz, "The Effects of Medicaid Expansion under the ACA: Updated Findings from a Literature Review," Kaiser Family Foundation (KFF), March 2020, http://files.kff.org/attachment/Report-The-Effects-of-Medicaid-Expansion-under-the-ACA-Updated-Findings-from-a-Literature-Review.pdf

18 JR Guardado and CK Kane, American Medical Association Division of Economic and Health Policy Research, "Competition in Health Insurance A Comprehensive Study of US Markets: 2020 Update," accessed December 17, 2020, https://www.ama-assn.org/system/files/2020-10/competition-health-insurance-us-markets.pdf

19 Louisiana Department of Health, Healthy Louisiana, "Medicaid Expansion Success Stories" accessed March 23, 2020, http://ldh.la.gov/index.cfm/page/2728

RESOURCES

OVERALL

America's Health Rankings at https://www.americashealthrankings.org/learn/reports/2020-annual-report

The 2020 KIDS COUNT Data Book: State Trends in Child Well-Being at https://www.aecf.org/resources/2020-kids-count-data-book/

Oklahoma State of the State's Health Report at https://stateofstateshealth.ok.gov/

Oklahoma Policy Issues at Oklahoma Policy Institute at okpolicy.org

INFANT MORTALITY RATE

Preparing for a Lifetime, Its Everyone's Responsibility at https://oklahoma.gov/health/family-health/improving-infant-outcomes.html

CANCER DEATHS

Information on how to prevent cancer or find it early at https://www.cdc.gov/cancer/dcpc/prevention/index.htm

Oklahoma Cancer Prevention and Control Plan at https://www.ok.gov/health2/documents/State%20Cancer%20Plan%202017-2022%20updated%20May%2010%202018.pdf

SUICIDE DEATH RATE

Suicide prevention lifeline at suicidepreventionlifeline.org or 1-800-273-TALK (8255)

DRUG DEATHS

Ways to dispose of prescription drugs at disposemymeds.org

Strategies to Prevent Opiate Abuse at https://www.cdc.gov/drugoverdose/pubs/featured-topics/evidence-based-strategies.htm

Preventing Adverse Childhood Experiences at https://www.cdc.gov/violenceprevention/pdf/preventingACES.pdf

Oklahoma Commission on Opiate Abuse at https://www.oag.ok.gov/ocoa

TOBACCO

Tobacco Helpline at okhelpline.com

Tobacco Stops with Me at stopswithme.com

Oklahoma State Tobacco Use Prevention and Cessation Plan at https://www.ok.gov/health2/documents/2019%20-%20OK%20State%20Plan%20for%20Tobacco%20Use%20Prevention%20%20Cessation.pdf

OBESITY

Tobacco Settlement Endowment Trust (TSET) Healthy Living Program at TSET.ok.gov

Obesity information at shapeyourfutureok.com

Get Fit Eat Smart Oklahoma Physical Activity and Nutrition State Plan at https://www.ok.gov/health2/documents/OKPAN__State__Plan.pdf

Robert Wood Johnson (RWJ) State of Childhood Obesity at https://stateofchildhoodobesity.org

Trust for America's Health (TFAH) Obesity at https://www.tfah.org/issue-details/obesity/

INCARCERATION RATE

Oklahoma Drug Courts at https://oklahoma.gov/odmhsas/substance-abuse/oklahoma-drug-and-mental-health-courts/adult-drug-court.html

Oklahoma Policy Institute at https://okpolicy.org/topic/justice-system/

Oklahomans for Criminal Justice Reform at prhttps://okjusticereform.org

Prison Policy Initiative at https://www.prisonpolicy.org

Oklahoma Justice Reform Task Force Report at https://www.ok.gov/dcs/searchdocs/app/manage__documents.php?att__id=22034

TEEN BIRTH RATE

Teen Pregnancy Prevention What Can Schools Do? at https://www.ok.gov/health2/documents/What%20You%20Can%20Do%20-%20Schools.pdf

Teen Pregnancy Prevention What Can Youth Serving Organizations Do? At https://www.ok.gov/health2/documents/What%20You%20Can%20Do%20-%20Youth%20Serving%20Organizations

Information on Teen Pregnancy at https://www.cdc.gov/teenpregnancy/index.htm

What Works: Sexual Health Education at https://www.cdc.gov/healthyyouth/whatworks/what-works-sexual-health-education.htm

Power to Decide Campaign to Prevent Unplanned Pregnancy at https://powertodecide.org

POVERTY

Oklahoma Poverty Issues at https://okpolicy.org/topic/poverty/

Effective Programs and Policies for Promoting Economic Well-Being at https://www.urban.org/research/publication/effective-programs-and-policies-promoting-economic-well-being

Children Living in High-Poverty, Low-Opportunity Neighborhoods at https://www.aecf.org/resources/children-living-in-high-poverty-low-opportunity-neighborhoods

EDUCATION

Building a Grad Nation Report at https://www.americaspromise.org/building-grad-nation-report

School-based health services at https://www.apha.org/-/media/files/pdf/sbhc/well__being__in__schools.ashx?la=en&hash=F54F7A314E6EB201C8B91F0EF8DDC673E6A35187

Oklahoma Report on the Future of Higher Education at https://www.okhighered.org/future/docs/final-report.pdf

Overlooked Value of Certificates and Associates Degrees at https://cew.
georgetown.edu/cew-reports/subba/

Launch Oklahoma Strategic Plan at https://oklahomaworks.gov/wp-
content/uploads/2017/04/Launch-OK-Strategic-Recommendations-2017.
pdf

UNINSURED

Benefits of Medicaid Expansion at https://okpolicy.org/medicaid-
expansion-ten-years-of-unparalleled-return-on-investment-improved-
outcomes/

Kaiser Family foundation: Key Facts About the Uninsured Population at
https://www.kff.org/uninsured/issue-brief/key-facts-about-the-uninsured-
population/

Acknowledgements

Oklahoma Pride: Working together for the Well-being of All Oklahomans fulfills a long-term dream to use art to illuminate health concerns in Oklahoma and identify actions that community and state leaders can take to improve the state's outcomes. This book would not have been possible without the wonderful team of advisers who spent countless hours in its design and creation.

We cannot say enough thanks to the students at the University of Oklahoma School of Visual Arts whose pictorial representations led the way: Emily Addington, Sydney Baird, Mikayla Baldwin, Paige Barber, Gabrielle Brann, Emilee Baumgarner, Andrea Burnsworth, Jillian Craighead, Jacob Cullum, Khoa Diep, Meghan Gaddy, Jacqueline Gilbert, Sidney Hallak, Peyton Hazel, Gloria Holland, Dixie Huckabay, Monica Kim, Crystal Kunze, Elizabeth Mahan, Jessica Mcginnis, Julie Nguyen, Brecke Pitt, Darby Sams, Brittany Young, and Nicholas Young.

There were many experts, representing diverse fields, who served as advisors for this book: Dr Terry Cline, Former Oklahoma Commissioner of Health; Gene Rainbolt, Chairman BancFirst Corporation; Kelly Dyer Fry, former editor and publisher at the *Oklahoman*; and Karen Thumann, Visual Communication Professor, Weitzenhoffer School of Fine Arts; and Jeffrey Dismukes, Chief Public Information Officer at the Oklahoma Department of Mental Health and Substance Abuse Services.

We are fortunate to have Jim Tolbert at Full Circle Press as the publisher of this book. The creative format is the work of Carl Brune.

We also want to acknowledge the following individuals for their significant contributions to this book, that of Dr. Gary Raskob, Dean of the Hudson College of Public Health who served as the overall editor of the book. He was joined by Dr. Sharon Neuwald as lead writer and Shawna Lawyer Struby and Marvin Smith who participated in the writing and editing of specific chapters.

Other individuals were significantly involved in the development of the *Oklahoma Pride*: They include VaLauna Grissom, Special Assistant at the Hudson College of Public Health; and Diane Sisemore, Senior Vice President at BancFirst.

You can see with this team that *Oklahoma Pride* exemplifies Mr. Rainbolt's motto "If you can get people to work together you can get more done." It is with that spirit of collective action that we present this book to you.

133